YOGA: AWAKENING THE INNER BODY

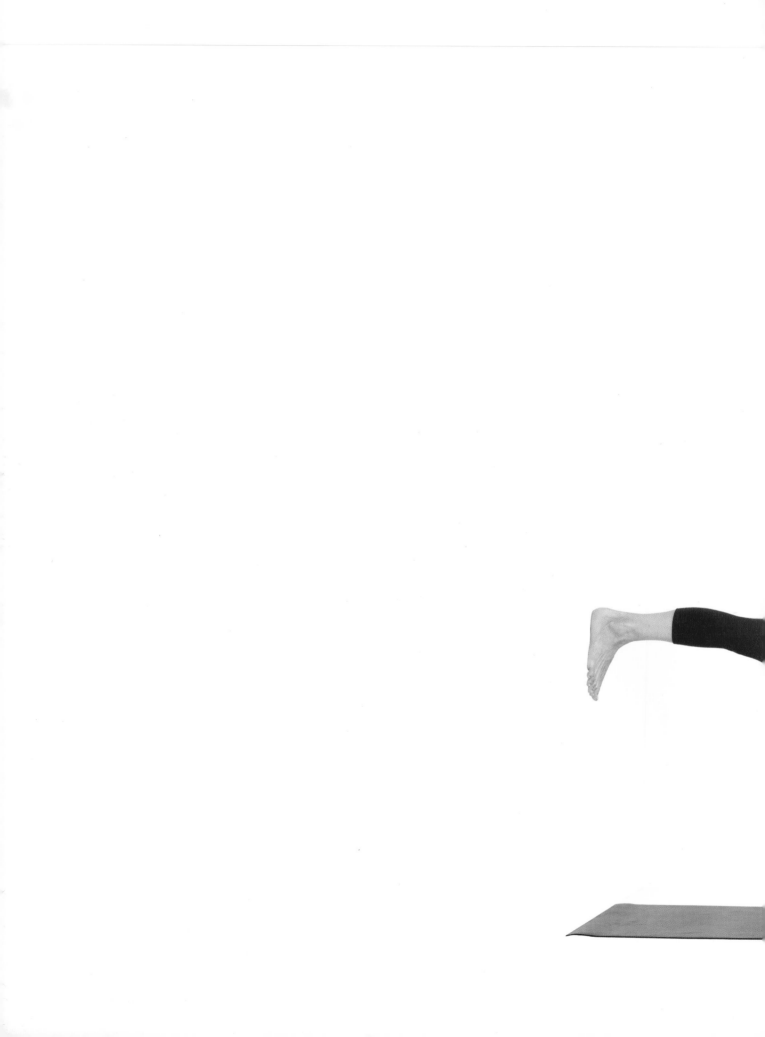

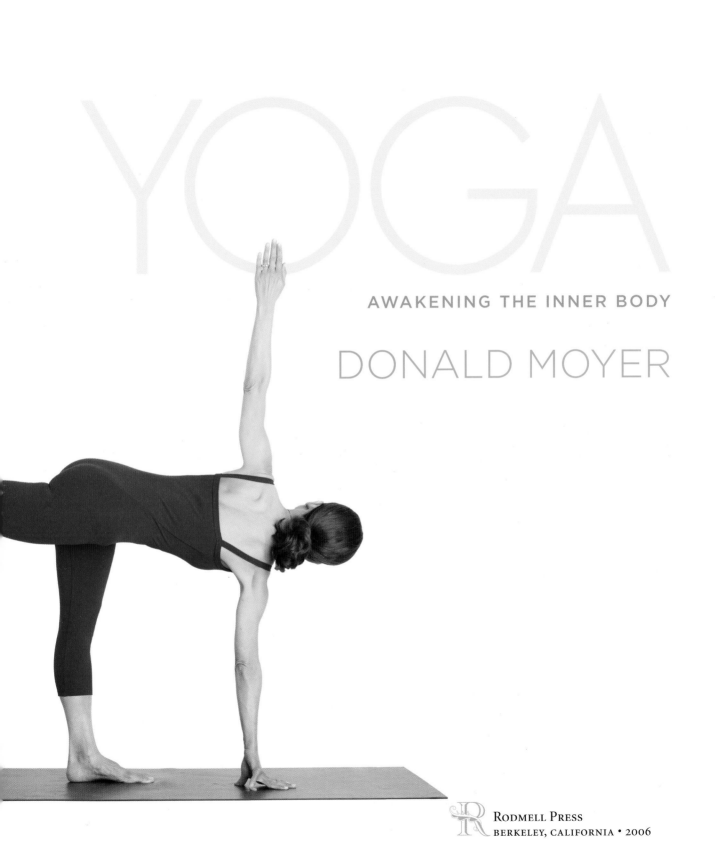

YOGA

AWAKENING THE INNER BODY

DONALD MOYER

RODMELL PRESS
BERKELEY, CALIFORNIA • 2006

Library of Congress Cataloging-in-Publication Data is available.

Printed in China
First Edition
ISBN-10: 1-930485-12-3
ISBN-13: 978-1-930485-12-9

12 11 10 09 08 07 06   1 2 3 4 5 6 7 8 9 10

Project Director
Linda Cogozzo

Copy Editor
Katherine L. Kaiser

Indexer
Ty Koontz

Cover and Text Design
Gopa & Ted2, Inc.

Cover and Interior Photographer
David Martinez

Illustrator
Krista McCurdy

Prepress
Charles Cunningham, Prepress Assembly, Inc.

Lithographer
Kwong Fat Offset Printing Co., Ltd.

Text set in Minion 10.25/15

Distributed by Publishers Group West

To Sri B. K. S. Iyengar, with gratitude

CONTENTS

Acknowledgments   ix

Preface by Susan Leigh Foster   xi

Introduction   1

PART ONE
FINDING INNER BALANCE

Chapter 1: Salamba Sarvangasana   13

Chapter 2: Salamba Sirsasana   37

PART TWO
THEMES AND VARIATIONS

Chapter 3: The Three Diaphragms   63

Chapter 4: Balance Your Sternum   93

Chapter 5: Collarbones, Kidneys, and Groins   121

Chapter 6: Align Your Shoulder Blades   149

Chapter 7: Stabilize Your Elbows   177

Chapter 8: Strengthen the Base of Your Neck   205

Glossary   233

Resources   235

About the Models   236

About the Author   237

From the Publisher   238

Index   239

ACKNOWLEDGMENTS

M
ANY PEOPLE have helped me in the writing of this book, but I want to express special feelings of gratitude to the following:

Sri B. K. S. Iyengar, for inspiring my practice and my teaching through his compassion, his genius, and his dedication to yoga;

My dear friend and mentor Maureen Carruthers, for first encouraging me to teach yoga, and for remaining my ideal of a sensitive, caring, and ultimately wise teacher;

Mary Lou Weprin, my incomparable codirector, and my other colleagues at The Yoga Room, especially Vicky Palmer, Barbara Papini, Gay White, Sandy Blaine, and Marie Hart, for working together selflessly to create an environment of mutual support and respect;

Workshop hosts Barbara Fergusson and Todd Jackson in Portland, Oregon; Annie Stocker, Wendy Groesbeck, and Chris Luboff in Seattle, Washington; Lynne Minton and Kathy Vasquez in Anchorage, Alaska; Candace Carey Satlak and Joseph Satlak in Boston; and Genny Kapuler in New York, for providing a forum for me to present the ideas in this book;

My students throughout the years, for helping me to understand what works and what doesn't work, and for teaching me to pay attention to individual needs and differences;

Susan Leigh Foster, for writing the preface in which her natural enthusiasm and keen intelligence shine through, and for offering many helpful suggestions for revising the text;

Shari Ser, P.T., for checking the accuracy of my anatomical details and for helping me to clarify my instructions;

Candace Carey Satlak and Joseph Satlak, for reading the manuscript meticulously, and for showing boundless patience, good humor, and dedication as models for this book;

Todd Jackson, for faithfully recording my seminars;

Craige Roberts, for generously archiving a work in progress;

Gopa and Veetam Campbell, at Gopa & Ted2, Inc., for encouraging people to use this book with their spacious and elegant design;

David Martinez, for creating the beautiful photographs in this book and for assembling an amazing crew: Mark Dawson (digital technician), France Dushane (hair and makeup), Malcolm Fearon (photographer's assistant), Aneata Ferguson (studio manager), Kristen Flammer (studio manager), and Jeff Mason (caterer);

Krista McCurdy, for breaking new ground with her inventive illustrations and for her delightful spirit;

Katherine L. Kaiser, for copyediting with care, and Ty Koontz, for creating the index;

Most important, Linda Cogozzo, copublisher at Rodmell Press, for encouraging me to write about yoga in the first place, and for guiding this book through its many stages. This project could not have succeeded without her tireless efforts, her high standards, and her expertise.

PREFACE BY SUSAN LEIGH FOSTER

WHEN I WALK INTO The Yoga Room, lodged in the annex of the Julia Morgan Center, a magnificent redwood building in Berkeley, California, designed by architect Julia Morgan, I feel lighter and more buoyant. The space resonates with the vibrant energy of alert practitioners whose exploration of yoga has been guided and encouraged by Donald Moyer. His gentle instructions, as practiced by many astute and diligent bodies throughout the years, have permeated the room, giving it a quiet jubilance.

In his teaching, Donald sets up class as a site of inquiry and investigation. He approaches each asana as if engaging with a proposition: "What if we focus on the lesser trochanter or the xiphoid process?" Instead of reciting a list of requirements, such as, *The leg is placed here* or *The chest is lifted there,* he asks students to focus their awareness on a particular area of the body and then to track its functioning through different poses. In this process, we learn the complexities of anatomy and the subtle integration of all parts of the body in each asana.

We also learn that there is no single right way to do a pose, but instead, that each body can realize its distinctive enactment of asana by reckoning with its history and structure. Some bodies have longer forearms or tighter hip joints; some work at the computer and others build houses. Some bodies need to adjust for these specificities by narrowing, others by widening; some by lengthening, others by firming; some by pressing, others by lifting. Thus, Donald's classes celebrate all different types of bodies and their variegated approaches to the dynamics, rather than the appearance, of asana.

Donald carefully chooses the descriptive language he uses in class so as to frame his instructions for poses in the positive. He seldom tells a student what *not* to do, nor does he invoke terms such as *lock, hit,* or *harden.* Instead, he guides the body toward the pose with directives such as *lengthen* or *expand* in order to encourage a student's increasing awareness of the body's needs and inclinations. This use of language also establishes a harmonious dialogue among awareness, will, and body: *How does it feel to do the pose this way? Or this way? Where does my effort come from? What kind of effort brings transformation?* As our bodies respond, we learn to listen.

Instead of "getting it right, finally," we learn from Donald's teaching to approach yoga as an ongoing unfolding of awareness. There is a limitless number of perspectives from which to examine each asana; there is an equally unlimited number of

SUSAN LEIGH FOSTER
is a choreographer,
scholar, and the author
of *Reading Dancing:
Bodies and Subjects in
Contemporary American
Dance* (University of
California Press) and
*Dances That Describe
Themselves: The Impro-
vised Choreography of
Richard Bull* (Wesleyan
University Press).

physicalities, who will engage poses uniquely. What matters is the daily invocation of a conversation within ourselves about how and what we are feeling, a conversation in which we experience how the work in the poses brings changes in mind and spirit as well as body.

Working with B. K. S. Iyengar, Donald gained a meticulous and profound under-standing of the body, and he also apprehended Iyengar's commitment to yoga as a continuous process of investigation. As many of his students know, Iyengar has revised his instructions and commentary about asana many times throughout the years, partly in response to the changing group of students he has instructed, and partly in response to his own deepening inquiry into yoga. That spirit of inquiry places a responsibility on each student to embrace the practice of yoga and find its meaning. Donald emphasizes this inquiry in his classes through the concentrated yet informal tone of his comments, his delight in the complexities of practice, his unas-suming willingness to entertain questions, his enthusiasm at students' growing aware-ness, his rigor, and his generosity.

Now, wonderfully, we have a book documenting Donald's approach and many of his rich insights into the process of practicing yoga. In it, you will find his careful attention to language and a down-to-earth yet precise set of metaphors for describing actions in the poses. Different chapters often refer to the same pose, examining its actions in different parts of the body. Comparing instructions for Adho Mukha Svanasana (Downward-Facing Dog Pose) in each chapter will give you a sense of the complexity of the pose. Don't worry if you initially have difficulty feeling the area referred to in the instructions. By repeatedly asking yourself to become aware of the three diaphragms, the kidneys, or the inner triceps, you will eventually establish a connection and learn to converse with them.

Often, physical practices are constructed around a struggle to create the "perfect" body or to ward off the effects of aging. Dancers, athletes, and many who aspire to physical fitness work against the impending debilitation of the body that is identified with growing older and toward some ideal body, basing their daily workouts on the assumption that "if there's no pain, there's no gain." In Donald's classes, I have learned that yoga is never painful. Like the Zen butcher whose knife always remained sharp because he knew just where to cut, Donald imparts a sense of how the pose can settle into the body as the body opens to receive it. The body feels nourished as the pose permeates it.

Especially at this moment in history, when bodies are being bullied into accom-plishing ever more exacting skills, it is crucial to imagine and implement alternative understandings of embodiment. Donald's approach to yoga offers a way to acquire a consciousness of the body as a limitless array of potential connections and interac-tions. And it posits awakening as an everyday, matter-of-fact process, the product of attentive listening to the world around and within us. That is why when I leave at the end of one of Donald's classes, I always feel both renewed and enlivened, as if I am growing, not older, but more aware.

INTRODUCTION

COULD NOT HAVE WRITTEN *Yoga: Awakening the Inner Body* without the teaching and inspiration I received from B.K.S. Iyengar. He taught me how to practice and how to teach, how to feel what was happening in my own body, and how to see and interpret what was happening in others. He gave me language and images for describing the internal experience of yoga, not just the mechanics. If there is anything of value in this book, it is due to his influence.

I began studying yoga with Penny Nield-Smith in London in 1971. Penny was one of Iyengar's first students in England, and a wonderful, inspiring teacher. She was also a dedicated social activist, and after class there was usually a petition to sign or a raffle ticket to purchase for some worthy cause. Angela Farmer, Kofi Busia, Bobby and Lindsay Clennell, and a host of other budding nonconformists started yoga with Penny as well.

In Penny's classes, we practiced all the standing poses each week, followed by inverted poses, backbends, twists, sitting poses, and Savasana (Figure 3.22). We didn't hold the poses long, but we sure did lots of them. When Iyengar came to town for his annual seminar, Penny stepped up the pace, and we practiced all the standing poses twice in the same amount of time.

In 1973, Penny invited me to observe Iyengar teach a class for his senior English students. This was my first glimpse of the great man. I sat cross-legged on the platform behind him, and watched in awe. I remember how he lined people up neatly in rows, and how he corrected their poses with astonishing speed and skill. *How does he know such things?* I asked myself in amazement. Toward the end of class, in a quieter mood, he described with exquisite detail how to work the tip of the big toe in Halasana (Figure 3.17). Not the whole big toe, just the tip!

In 1974, I moved to Vancouver, British Columbia, and with the encouragement of my friend and mentor Maureen Carruthers, began teaching yoga. I had no training whatsoever to teach, and relied solely on my memory of Penny's classes, and her clear and straightforward instructions. In fact, for the first two years of teaching, I repeated everything Penny had said—including her jokes and her pithy sayings.

The first time I studied with Iyengar in India, in January 1976, a year after the opening of the Ramamani Iyengar Memorial Yoga Institute in Pune, I was not prepared for his extraordinary use of the English language. For one thing, he referred to obscure parts of the body, not generally found in *Gray's Anatomy*, such as "the chips of the knees" and "the eyes of the chest." He had created a language of awareness based not on how he saw the body from the outside, but on how he experienced the body from the inside.

For another thing, his syntax was so elliptical and ambiguous that it defied logical analysis. During class, I knew what he was saying as he was saying it, because my body responded so readily to his words; but after class, when everyone had a different interpretation of what he had said, my understanding seemed to evaporate. In the end, it didn't matter. He spoke to our bodies, not to our brains.

Finally, Iyengar's teaching changed from day to day. Whereas my first teacher, Penny, repeated the same instructions class after class, week after week, until they were printed indelibly in my brain, Iyengar never taught the same pose in the same way twice. Each class had a different theme and a different focus. It was like the Japanese film *Rashomon*: every part of the body had its own version of the story to tell.

Starting with my first intensive, I took copious notes after every class. I began by listing all the poses we had practiced that day, in the sequence we had practiced them. At the top of the page, I briefly noted Iyengar's theme for the day: "intercostal muscles," "the chips of the knees," or the ever-baffling and mysterious "the object becomes the subject and the subject becomes the object." Next I wrote down everything I could remember that Iyengar had said during class, and everything that my friends and companions could remember as well. My notes filled many looseleaf binders, but they proved virtually unusable. I could not recapture in my home practice what I had not experienced in my own body.

As I mentioned, I attended my first intensive in Pune in January 1976. I worked with Iyengar again in Berkeley in May 1976, and decided to move to California. I returned to India in January 1977 and for a longer period from October to December of that year. I continued to document my classes with Iyengar relentlessly.

By the end of 1977, the sheer volume of my notes compelled me to reconsider my approach. Instead of writing down everything I remembered (or misremembered), I went down the list, pose by pose, and asked myself, *What did you experience in the pose today that felt new or meaningful?* With this new method, my notes became radically shorter—but much more coherent.

When I returned to California, I began keeping a journal of my yoga practice in a stenographer's pad that I labeled *Asana Daybook*. I did not write in this journal every day, but only when something occurred in my practice that I wanted to remember and to explore further. These notes were brief and cryptic, but the very act of writing them down helped me to train my mind—first by observing what happened in my body, and then by describing my experience. This process brought continuity to my practice and taught me patience.

My next visit to Pune, in October 1979, marked a turning point in my life. I realized on the first day of the intensive that my understanding had taken a quantum leap. Both my body and my mind were attuned to Iyengar's instructions. I believe that Iyengar recognized this change in me as well. For the next two days, he watched me like a hawk, constantly barking out my name and challenging me in my poses. For me, this rite of passage brought a deep sense of awakening and validation of my way of being. From that time on, I felt I could trust in my own experience of the poses.

In the practice of yoga, as in any other spiritual practice, there are many kinds of awakening. There is the sudden awakening that comes out of the blue and is filled with the wonder of discovery. I remember the burst of joy and the sense of liberation I felt after my very first class with Penny.

Then comes the everyday form of awakening—the quiet *Ahas!* the small but significant insights, the brief flashes of understanding—which, added one to another, mark the incremental growth of awareness, the way a plant forms a bud before it comes into flower.

Further along comes the awakening to your own nature, to your own potential, the rite of passage that confirms that even though you may benefit from the guidance of a teacher, nevertheless, you have the courage, the integrity, and the sense of responsibility to find your own way out of the labyrinth. This stage of the journey initiates the awakening of the inner body, when the body reveals its secrets, one by one, just as a flower unfolds, petal by petal.

▶
DEFINING THE INNER BODY

What do I mean by the "inner body"? For me, the inner body involves every aspect of a person's being: the anatomical, the physiological, the mental, and the spiritual.

Surface Muscles versus Deeper Muscles. At the anatomical level, the large external muscles that wrap the surface of the body belong to the outer body, whereas the deeper, more intrinsic muscles correspond to the inner body. When you practice yoga using your external muscles, your movements are strong but effortful. As you learn to release the grip of the surface muscles and engage the intrinsic muscles, you move deeper into the pose, with much less effort.

In the practice of *asana* (yoga poses), the surface muscles and the deeper muscles should be properly balanced to reduce tension and maintain healthy alignment. The sequence in Chapter 8, for example, explores the reciprocal relationship between the trapezius (superficial muscles of the neck and shoulders) and the splenius (deeper muscles that support the cervical spine).

Anatomical Body versus Physiological Body. In simplest terms, the anatomical, or outer, body refers to the skeletal system of muscles and bones, whereas the physiological, or inner, body relates to the internal organs, including the liver, stomach, heart, lungs, and kidneys, and to the physiological processes of the body. Thus, the outer body is the structural, or mechanical, body, and the inner body is the energetic, or subtle, body.

The anatomical body and the physiological body must be properly aligned with each other to optimize the movement of your spine and the flow of energy. For example, the practice sequence in Chapter 5 explores the spatial relationship between your kidneys and your rib cage. If your rib cage is attempting a backbend but your kidneys are engaged in a forward bend, or if your rib cage moves into a forward bend but your kidneys are still in a backbend mode, the movement of your spine will be compromised.

The Active Mind versus the Reflective Mind. At the mental level, the active mind represents the outer world of thinking, doing, and acting; the reflective mind stands for the inner world of feeling, sensing, and responding.

For the practice of yoga to be nourishing and creative, there must be a dialogue between the active, or intentional, mind and the reflective, or receptive, mind. If you are ruled by the active mind, your practice becomes forced and mechanical because you never listen to your body: you treat it like a machine. If you are ruled by the reflective mind, your practice becomes formless and inert, and loses its sense of purpose.

In practicing with this book, I hope you will follow my instructions, but not take them too literally. Ask yourself frequently, *How does it feel?* If an adjustment feels good to you—if your pose feels lighter, if your spine lengthens, or if your breathing feels easier—take this as positive.

If an adjustment doesn't seem to work—if you feel increased tension, if you feel more discomfort, or if your breathing feels constricted—your body is telling you not to proceed. In this case, ask yourself why the instruction didn't work. Are you overcorrecting? Are you clinging to an old idea of what the pose should look like? How can you modify, or adapt, the instruction to make it work for you? In this way, you will find your own voice and your own way of being in the pose.

The Ego versus the Self. At the spiritual level, the ego is your psychological means for coping with the outer world and creating a semblance of rational order. The self is the monitor of your inner world, feeding you images and intuitions as elusive as a mirage in the desert, guiding you toward an unforeseen goal.

Your challenge at this level of being is to give up control and loosen the grip of the ego. In your yoga practice, be willing to give up everything you thought you knew: every tradition, every authority, every cherished notion. Be willing to question every idea about alignment and every principle of movement, and follow your practice wherever it leads, day after day, with courage and faith.

The awakening of the inner body can be cultivated and prolonged so that it leads to a lifetime of discovery. But there is another form of awakening that is beyond your control. In yoga tradition, this final stage of awakening, or enlightenment, is known as *samadhi*. In samadhi, body, mind, and ego drop away. You go beyond sensing and feeling, beyond thoughts and words, and beyond all division between inner and outer, self and other, and experience only the unity of all being.

There are no methods or techniques that can guarantee this state of grace. You can only prepare yourself as best you can. As Krishnamurti writes in *Freedom from the Known,*

> Up to now we can describe, explain, but no words or explanation can open the
> door. What will open the door is daily awareness and attention—awareness of
> how we speak, what we say, how we walk, what we think. It is like cleaning a
> room and keeping it in order. Keeping the room in order is important in one
> sense but *totally* unimportant in another. There must be order in the room but

order will not open the door or the window. What will open the door is not your volition or your desire. You cannot possibly invite the *other*. All that you can do is to keep the room in order, which is to be virtuous for itself, not for what it will bring. To be sane, rational, orderly. Then perhaps, if you are lucky, the window will open and the breeze will come in.[1]

▶ PLANNING YOUR HOME PRACTICE

Yoga: Awakening the Inner Body is intended for students and teachers who want to develop their awareness and deepen their home practice. To benefit from the sequences in this book, you will, ideally, practice a minimum of three times a week for at least an hour each time, in addition to any classes you may be attending.

A home yoga practice can be an enhancement to your life, a time you spend with yourself to nourish and revitalize yourself. If you expect too much of yourself in terms of your practice, it will turn into another burden or chore and you may give up completely. Before embarking on a home practice, consider carefully how much time you have available each day. Make a list or chart of your working hours, household tasks, and family responsibilities, and see how you can reasonably fit a yoga practice into your life.

Choose a clean, quiet space for your practice area, preferably with a bare floor and an accessible wall. When you practice, turn off your telephone or switch on your answering machine. Let your friends and family know this is your quiet time, and you are not to be disturbed.

Ideally, you will not eat for at least 2 hours before practicing. If this is not possible, eat something light, such as fruit, but stop eating 1 hour before doing yoga.

Wear clothing that does not restrict the movement of your legs or pelvis. Shorts and T-shirt, leotard and tights, or sweat clothes are fine. Practice barefoot to enhance your balance and sensitize your feet.

▶ GATHER YOUR PROPS

Before you begin your practice, gather all your props. Initially, you may feel some resistance to using props, but once you learn to listen to your body, you will discover that props can take you deeper and help you feel better in a pose. Used effectively, props can do the following:

- ▶ make difficult poses more accessible
- ▶ relieve pain and discomfort

1. J. Krishnamurti, *Freedom from the Known* (New York: Harper & Row, 1969), 33.

- ▶ prevent injury
- ▶ release tension and provide support
- ▶ maintain proper alignment
- ▶ create space in the joints
- ▶ enhance movement
- ▶ develop awareness and understanding

The downside to using props is that you can become dependent on them and not practice to your full potential. You can avoid this pitfall by practicing each pose once with a prop and then once without. When you practice without a prop, try to recreate the same movement and alignment that the prop made possible. In this way, you will not only develop your understanding of the pose but also reduce your reliance on the prop. Even if you use a prop primarily to prevent pain or injury, every few weeks try the pose briefly without a prop and cautiously measure your progress.

Here's what you will need:

ONE OR TWO NONSKID MATS. A nonskid mat provides a smooth, firm surface and allows you to practice standing poses without slipping. A standard nonskid mat is 24 inches wide, 68 inches long, and approximately 1/8 inch thick, although thicker mats are available.

I recommend having one nonskid mat for standing and lying on, and another for rolling, folding, and using as an additional support. If you have an old mat that needs replacing, cut away the worn-out sections and save the remnants for making smaller props.

FOUR TO SIX FOLDED BLANKETS. You will need four to six wool or cotton blankets, primarily for Salamba Sarvangasana (Figure 1.1). Blankets measure about 60 inches wide and 80 inches long, but for yoga purposes are usually folded four times into a rectangle that is approximately 20 inches wide and 30 inches long. Four blankets are more than adequate for most people, but you may need five or six for Salamba Sarvangasana if you have problems with your neck.

Throughout this book, the phrase *folded blanket* or *standard folded blanket* refers to a blanket folded to 20 inches wide and 30 inches long. On specified occasions, the folded blanket is folded again: in half lengthwise (10 inches wide and 30 inches long), in half crosswise (15 inches wide and 20 inches long), or in thirds crosswise (10 inches wide and 20 inches long).

ONE ROUND BOLSTER. A round bolster is ideal for restorative, or resting, poses, and can be used in a variety of ways. A round bolster is typically about 2 feet long and 9 inches in diameter.

If you do not have a round bolster, you can roll two folded blankets in the shape of a bolster. Starting from the narrow end, roll the first blanket tightly. Then wrap the second blanket around the first one as snugly as possible.

ONE CHAIR. A metal folding chair is most convenient for yoga practice and is easily stored. If you cannot locate a folding chair, you can use a wooden straight-backed chair, provided that it has no rollers.

TWO TO FIVE BLOCKS. Yoga blocks are made from a variety of materials (chiefly wood or foam) and come in different sizes (usually 3½ inches wide, 5½ inches high, and 9 inches long, or 4 inches wide, 6 inches high, and 9 inches long). Wooden blocks are sturdier and more expensive; foam blocks are lighter and cheaper. Whatever variety you choose, make sure you have a pair of blocks that are identical in size and shape.

You can manage with only two blocks, but I prefer having four: one pair of wooden blocks and one pair of foam blocks. I use wooden blocks when I need greater stability, such as in Setu Bandhasana with Blocks Under the Sacrum (Figure 8.20), but foam blocks when a softer, yielding surface feels more comfortable, as in Uttanasana (Figure 3.7) with a block between the knees.

You will need five blocks only if you practice Salamba Sirsasana with Blocks at the Wall (Figure 2.16a), as described in Chapter 2.

Throughout this book, the phrase *place your block flat* means to lay your block with the largest surface parallel to the floor; *place your block on its side* means to position your block so that it rests on its long, narrow side; and *place your block on end* means to stand your block upright on its smallest surface.

ONE STRAP WITH A BUCKLE. A yoga strap with a buckle is usually about 1½ inches wide, and 6, 8, or 10 feet long. The 6-foot length is adequate for most students, but if you are taller, you may need a longer strap.

ONE WEDGE. A wedge, or slantboard, can be placed under your hands to reduce pressure on your wrists or under your heels to support your feet. Numerous other ways to use a wedge are suggested throughout this book.

A wedge measures about 6 inches wide and 20 inches long, the slope diminishing gradually from 2 inches high on the thick edge down toward the thin edge. Most students find a foam wedge most convenient, but wooden ones are also available.

ONE FACECLOTH. A facecloth can be folded or rolled to create a small prop when needed. When rolling a facecloth, use rubber bands to hold the roll in place.

TWO HAND TOWELS. A hand towel can be folded or rolled to create a slightly larger prop than a facecloth. When rolling a hand towel, use rubber bands to hold the roll in place.

The following props are optional:

ONE TIMER. An electronic timer with a soft beep is useful for timing your poses, especially Salamba Sirsasana (Figure 2.1), Salamba Sarvangasana (Figure 1.1), and sitting forward bends.

ONE TENNIS BALL. Chapter 2 describes how to use a tennis ball in Salamba Sirsasana (Figure 2.1) to maintain the cup of your hands.

▶
READING AND USING THIS BOOK

Yoga: Awakening the Inner Body is divided into two parts. "Part I: Finding Inner Balance" contains individual chapters on Salamba Sarvangasana and Salamba Sirsasana to help you establish your level of practice of these quintessential inverted poses. "Part II: Themes and Variations" consists of six practice sequences: each sequence focuses on a different theme related to the upper body. The appendix contains a glossary, resource listing, and index for easy reference.

"Part I: Finding Inner Balance." The first two chapters are divided into three sections. The opening section describes how to practice Salamba Sarvangasana (Chapter 1) and Salamba Sirsasana (Chapter 2) in systematic detail:

- ▶ how to choose and arrange the props you need, depending on your body type
- ▶ how to come into the pose effectively
- ▶ how to check your alignment once you are in the pose
- ▶ how to adjust for imbalances in the pose
- ▶ how to come out of the pose safely

Read this opening section carefully, even if you are practicing an alternative to Salamba Sarvangasana or Salamba Sirsasana. Many of the instructions and directions for the complete pose are helpful for the variations and alternatives.

The second section addresses beginners and those who are not yet practicing the final version of Salamba Sarvangasana or Salamba Sirsasana. This section opens with "Cautions and Considerations," to be read and reviewed by everyone. "Advice for Beginners" gives general guidelines for choosing alternatives and outlines the progression from variations to the complete pose. "Variations and Alternatives" presents these poses in full detail.

The last section, "Practice Suggestions," gives different ways for timing and organizing your practice, including guidelines for sequencing Salamba Sarvangasana and Salamba Sirsasana by taking into account the time of day, your particular body type, and the other poses you are practicing that day.

Read Part I carefully to determine what props you need for Salamba Sarvangasana and Salamba Sirsasana, and to establish your basic level of practice before proceeding to Part II. The practice sequences in Part II will help you refine your understanding and deepen your practice of these two essential poses. If you encounter any problems with Salamba Sarvangasana or Salamba Sirsasana, review Chapters 1 and 2 thoroughly to help identify the source of your concern.

"Part II: Themes and Variations." This part consists of six chapters, each focusing on a different part of the upper body: the three diaphragms, the sternum, the collarbones, the shoulder blades, the elbows, and the neck. (In a second volume, I hope to cover aspects of the lower body: the feet, the knees, the hamstrings and calves, the groins, the tailbone, and the sacrum.) Each chapter begins with an anatomical introduction that establishes the theme to be explored in the subsequent practice sequence, and discusses questions of alignment.

The practice sequences contain a variety of poses, including standing poses, backbends, twists, inverted poses, sitting forward bends, and *pranayama* (yoga breathing). Each sequence gives you the opportunity to explore a particular part of your body and experience how it responds differently in different poses. For instance, you understand in your own body why your collarbones need to move one way in backbends but the opposite way in forward bends.

Each pose is identified by its Sanskrit name and the English equivalent, and the following are discussed:

- ▶ props (and optional props, when necessary)
- ▶ benefits and cautions
- ▶ how to move into the pose
- ▶ how to check your alignment
- ▶ how to adjust in the pose
- ▶ how to come out of the pose
- ▶ additional practice notes (when necessary)
- ▶ a list of related poses (when applicable)

Some poses are repeated in different chapters, but each time the pose is described from a different perspective, so that you learn new movements and deepen your awareness. (Suggestions on how to use props for beginning students or those with special needs are placed in parentheses to indicate they are optional, and not intended for all practitioners.)

Each chapter concludes with a list of the poses described in the chapter for your convenience in practicing.

In Part II of *Yoga: Awakening the Inner Body,* you can either work with the chapters sequentially, or you can start with the chapter that seems most relevant and interesting to you. For instance, you may be curious about the movement of your shoulder blades. Or you may want a practice sequence to help you strengthen your neck. Or perhaps you are coming to terms with a broken collarbone. Whatever your interest, begin with the chapter that addresses your particular needs.

With each chapter, read the introduction carefully *before* you begin the practice sequence. If you are unfamiliar with the introductory material, read it two or three times, if necessary, and study the photos and drawings to develop your kinesthetic sense.

When you begin the practice sequence, work with a few poses at a time until you understand the theme of the chapter. This may take a few days or even weeks. Eventually, you will be able to practice the entire sequence in an hour to an hour and a half. Once you have mastered the basic sequence, you can begin to include the related poses.

When following the instructions in this book, remember to use your common sense. If I suggest something that causes discomfort or pain or doesn't feel right, please don't persist. My primary purpose in writing this book is not to dictate how you do the poses, but to share with you a way of practicing that deepens your awareness and understanding.

Even if my words help you, you cannot depend on them alone. Each of us needs to reinterpret what we experience in our own language. This is especially true for teachers, so that we can pass on the gift to those who follow. At the first anniversary celebrations of the Ramamani Iyengar Memorial Yoga Institute in Pune in January 1976, I remember Iyengar's closing words: "In my end is your beginning." These words still reverberate for me more than thirty years later.

Please take this work and carry it one step further.

PART 1:

Finding Inner Balance

1 SALAMBA SARVANGASANA

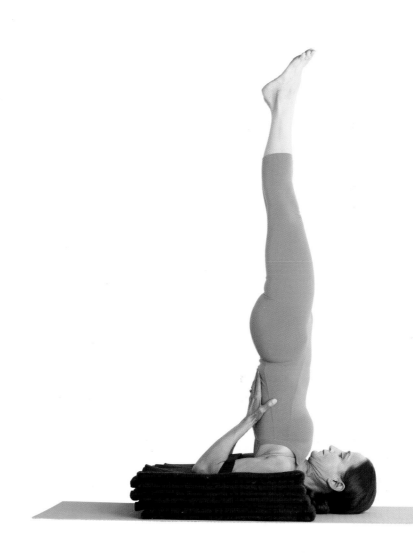

SALAMBA SARVAGANSANA (Figure 1.1) is generally known to yoga practitioners as Shoulderstand. *Salamba* means "supported": the arms and hands are used to support the torso. *Sarvangasana* means literally, "whole body pose," because it relieves so many common ailments, and restores both physical and mental vitality. In particular, the gentle pressure of the chin lock on the front of the throat increases the circulation of blood to this area, and thus stimulates the thyroid and parathyroid glands located here. The thyroid gland, through the release of hormones, regulates the flow of energy for all our bodily functions. Thus, Salamba Sarvangasana has a calming effect on the mind and releases the healing energies of the body.

CAUTION

If you have never practiced Salamba Sarvangasana (Figure 1.1) or don't know if the pose is appropriate for you, please read "Cautions and Considerations" p. 24) and "Advice for Beginners" (p. 25) before proceeding.

SALAMBA SARVANGASANA
SHOULDERSTAND

PROPS
• 1 to 6 blankets

OPTIONAL PROPS
• 1 nonskid mat
• 1 facecloth or hand towel
• 1 folded nonskid mat
• 1 bolster
• 1 to 2 straps
• 1 bolster, chair, or wall

▶
ESTABLISHING YOUR FOUNDATION

How many blankets you need for Salamba Sarvangasana and how to arrange them depends on your body type. This section helps you choose the foundation that is right for you by taking into account your degree of flexibility, the shape of your shoulders, and the curve of your neck.

Arranging Your Blankets. For your safety and comfort in practicing Salamba Sarvangasana, I recommend that you use a stack of two to four folded blankets under your shoulders and upper arms to help you lift higher onto your shoulders, create space between the back of your neck and the floor, and reduce any pressure on your head, eyes, or ears.

Folding Your Blankets. Start by folding each blanket in half four times so that it measures approximately 30 inches long by 20 inches wide. (Throughout this book, I

facing page:
1.1
Salamba Sarvangasana

use the phrase *folded blanket* to refer to a blanket folded in this way.) Fold your blankets neatly so that you have a smooth surface wide enough and deep enough to support your shoulders, upper arms, and elbows.

Stacking Your Blankets. Stack your blankets by aligning the folded edges of the blankets, not the open, ragged edges. (Your shoulders will be placed at the folded edge of the stack.) To create a firm foundation, most people place their blankets one directly on top of the other, forming a vertical edge. However, if your blankets slip and slide over each other as you come up into the pose, you may prefer a stepped-edge arrangement, where each successive blanket is placed ½ to 1 inch farther back from the edge of the one below it.

Supporting Your Head. Place your stack of blankets on a carpet or thick pad, so that your head is not pressing directly onto the hard floor. If you place your blankets on a nonskid mat, you may find that your hair sticks to the mat and you are unable to move the base of your skull away from your shoulders. In this case, spread a facecloth or hand towel under your head so that you can release the base of your skull and lengthen your neck.

How Many Blankets? How many blankets you need for Salamba Sarvangasana depends on the flexibility of your shoulders and the curve of your neck. As a general rule, you need higher blankets if your shoulders are tighter, and lower blankets if they are more flexible. For most people, two to four blankets is the optimum number. However, some students may require more than four blankets because of neck problems or spinal imbalances, while others can practice comfortably with one blanket or no blanket at all.

If you are not sure how many blankets to use for Salamba Sarvangasana, start with three blankets, and then, if necessary, either add or take away blankets. Ideally, your stack of blankets should be high enough so that your weight is distributed evenly between your elbows and your shoulders. If your weight drops onto your elbows and your shoulders are not in contact with your support, you need an additional blanket or two to come higher onto your shoulders.

On the other hand, if your weight rests on your shoulders but your elbows have no support, you can probably reduce the number of blankets you use, unless you have problems with your neck. If your shoulders are flexible but you need to use higher blankets to avoid discomfort in your neck, make sure that your elbows have adequate support. If your elbows lift away from your blankets, use a folded nonskid mat or other support under your elbows. Be sure to place this additional lift under your elbows only, not under your upper arms.

(For a further discussion on the height of your blankets, see "More About Blankets" later in this chapter.)

Sloping Shoulders. If you have sloping shoulders, rather than square-set shoulders, you may need to arrange your blankets in a different way for Salamba Sarvangasana (Figure 1.2).

If you have square-set shoulders, the weight of your body rests naturally on your outer shoulders and arms when you practice Salamba Sarvangasana, not on the base

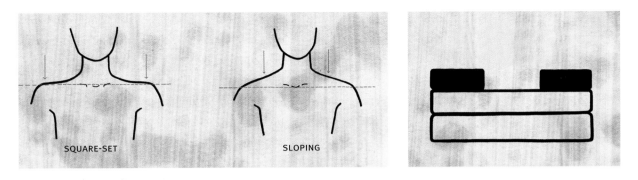

SQUARE-SET   SLOPING

1.2
Square-set and Sloping Shoulders

1.3
Blanket Arrangement for Sloping Shoulders

of your neck. However, if you have shoulders that slope at a steep angle, your outer shoulders may not be in contact with the blanket, causing all your weight to fall on the trapezius muscles at the base of your neck. In this case, you may feel pressure on your seventh cervical vertebra (C7) or discomfort in your neck, and with prolonged practice of Salamba Sarvangasana, the trapezius muscles at the base of your neck may become thick and swollen.

You can understand better how this happens by measuring the distance between the line of your outer shoulders and your C7. If you have square-set shoulders, your C7 is usually an inch or so above this line. If you have sloping shoulders, your C7 may be as much as 3 or 4 inches above the line of your outer shoulders. If you have sloping shoulders and practice Salamba Sarvangasana with your blankets laid flat, the pressure on the base of your neck will eventually cause your C7 and upper thoracic vertebrae to protrude.

To accommodate sloping shoulders, try the following arrangement of blankets in Salamba Sarvangasana. First, stack one or two folded blankets in the usual way as your foundation. Then take two more folded blankets, fold them each in half again, and place them parallel to each other on your foundation blankets with a groove between them that measures 4 to 6 inches. When you lie down, place your outer shoulders on the raised blankets, and let the muscles at the base of your neck rest in the groove so that they can release and lengthen. The groove will also help diminish the pressure you feel on your C7 and upper thoracic spine (Figure 1.3).

When you arrange your blankets in this way, make sure that the two raised blankets are identical in thickness. You may need to adjust the height of your raised blankets or the width of the groove. Remember that the raised blankets are intended to provide support for your outer shoulders, and space for your trapezius muscles and neck to relax.

With a Bolster Under Your Pelvis. If you use three or more blankets for Salamba Sarvangasana or if you have difficulty swinging your legs overhead, place a bolster in line with your blankets, so that your pelvis and legs are on the same level as your rib cage when you lie on your blankets.

▶ Assessing the Curve of Your Neck

Before placing your shoulders on your blanket, take a few moments to locate your C7 and assess the curve of your neck. Stand in Tadasana (Figure 3.3) with the crown of your head in line with your tailbone and lengthen your spine. To find your C7, first, place your fingers on the knobby protruberance at the base of your neck. Then look up at the ceiling. If your fingers are on C7, the bone will slide forward slightly. If not, you are pressing the first thoracic vertebra (T1). In this case, move your fingers up to the next level and try again.

Once you have found C7, does it lie flat, does it project slightly, or is it prominent? Does the flesh around C7 feel firm and resilient, or thick and swollen? (If the flesh at the base of your neck feels thick and swollen, your C7 is probably stressed. See "Sloping Shoulders" earlier in this chapter.)

The alignment of your C7 is crucial because it marks the transition between your cervical spine and your thoracic spine. If your C7 is displaced, your head and neck cannot balance properly on your upper back, and you are more vulnerable to neck injuries. (See Chapter 8 for ways to realign your C7 and strengthen the deeper muscles of your neck.)

Now run your fingertips up and down the center of your neck, and feel how the spinous processes of your cervical spine are aligned. Does the curve of your neck feel natural, contracted, or reversed? If you are uncertain about the shape of your neck, ask your teacher or an experienced friend for help (Figure 1.4).

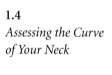

1.4
Assessing the Curve of Your Neck

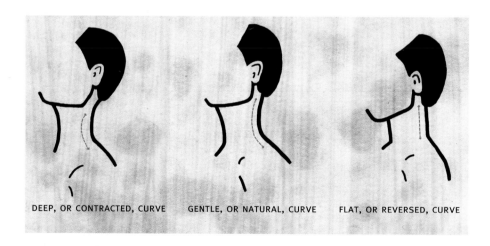

DEEP, OR CONTRACTED, CURVE   GENTLE, OR NATURAL, CURVE   FLAT, OR REVERSED, CURVE

Natural Curve. If your cervical spine curves gently inward and the crown of your head is parallel with the ceiling, your neck has a gentle, or natural, curve. In this case, place your shoulders so that C7 is perched at the very edge of your blankets when you are in Salamba Sarvangasana. (If your C7 is too far on the blanket, you may feel discomfort at the base of your neck.)

Contracted Curve. If your cervical spine moves deeply inward and your chin tilts up toward the ceiling, the curve of your neck is overarched and contracted. In this case, continue to place your C7 near the edge of your blankets, but use higher blankets under your shoulders to avoid straining the tight muscles and ligaments at the back of your neck.

(If, in addition to a contracted curve, your C7 is prominent, and the flesh at the base of your neck feels thick and swollen, check the shape of your shoulders, as described in "Sloping Shoulders.")

Flat or Reversed Curve. If your cervical spine has lost its natural curve and feels flat, or if the curve of your cervical spine has reversed and moves outward rather than inward, placing your C7 at the edge of your blanket would not be helpful. In this case, when your neck hangs freely in the space between your blankets and the floor, there is no support to prevent your cervical spine from bowing farther out of shape.

If the curve of your neck is flat or reversed, place more of your neck on your blanket, so that your cervical spine is supported. The edge of your blanket should come halfway up your cervical spine, or even higher, but should not press on the base of your skull. Take some time to find the placement that feels most comfortable to you.

▶ COMING INTO SALAMBA SARVANGASANA

Once you have arranged your blankets to suit your particular body type, you are ready to consider how to move into the pose. In my experience, many students come into Salamba Sarvangasana by narrowing their shoulders and squeezing their shoulder blades toward the spine. This movement tightens the trapezius muscles, strains the neck, and restricts the lift of the upper back.

As an alternative, I recommend that you widen your shoulders and lift your shoulder blades away from the floor to come higher onto your shoulders. You will learn this basic adjustment much more readily if you begin by using a strap around your arms when practicing this pose. Once you are proficient at lifting your shoulder blades with the aid of the strap, you can practice Salamba Sarvangasana without the strap.

Using a Strap on Your Arms. Make a loop with your strap that is approximately the width of your shoulders. Hang the loop around one of your elbows, and lie down with your shoulders at the edge of your blankets. Lift your pelvis a few inches, and hook your other arm into the strap behind your back, so that the strap rests just above your elbows. Then extend your arms along the sides of your body with your palms facing down. With an inhalation, broaden your shoulders against the blanket, and lengthen the back of your arms. With an exhalation, swing your legs overhead and lower your feet to the floor in Halasana with a Strap (Figure 1.5). If your hamstrings are tight, rest your feet on a bolster, chair, or wall.

In Halasana with a Strap, relax your shoulders and widen your collarbones. Turn your palms toward the floor to avoid hyperextending your elbows. Then press your upper arms out against the strap, and lengthen the back of your arms from your shoulders toward your elbows. At the same time, firm the muscles of your back armpits, and lift your shoulder blades away from the floor. Repeat this adjustment three or four times, until your shoulder blades are lifted to the maximum.

Adjusting Your Strap. When using a strap around your arms, make sure that it is neither too loose nor too tight. If your strap is too loose, it will not give you sufficient support. If your strap is too tight, your neck will feel strained and your shoulders narrow and constricted. Adjust the width of your strap so that you have the freedom to widen your shoulders and lift your shoulder blades.

Placing Your Hands on Your Back. When you have adjusted your rib cage and shoulder blades in Halasana with a Strap, place your hands flat on your back with your palms broad and your fingers pointing toward your waist. Then raise your legs toward the ceiling to come into Salamba Sarvangasana, and let your rib cage rest lightly against your hands (Figure 1.6).

Once in Salamba Sarvangasana, check that you have placed your hands evenly so that one hand is not higher than the other on your rib cage or farther out to the side. Observe the balance between your inner and your outer hands. If your weight falls more heavily on your inner hands (thumb sides) than on your outer hands (little-finger sides), your elbows are probably slipping out. To bring your elbows closer to the sides of your body, press the outer edges of your hands into your rib cage, and lengthen your fourth and fifth fingers toward your waist.

Finally, create a balance between the heels of your hands and the bottom knuckles of your fingers. If your weight falls more heavily on the heels of your hands, press the bottom knuckles (especially the knuckles at the base of your index fingers) firmly into your rib cage, and lengthen through your fingers. The more you can balance your hands in Salamba Sarvangasana, the more you balance the pose.

When you place your hands on your back with your fingers pointing toward your waist, you encourage your spine to lift vertically. There is a direct line of energy from your elbows through your forearms, hands, and fingers that continues upward through your spine and legs.

1.5
Halasana with a Strap

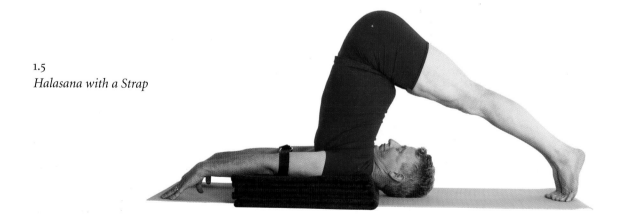

If, on the contrary, you place your hands on your back with your fingers pointing toward your spine, this flow of energy is disrupted. In this position, instead of lifting your spine, you tend to push your lower rib cage forward with the force of your hands, putting increased pressure on your neck and head. Furthermore, your elbows and upper arms slide away from your torso in response to the lateral movement of your hands. Not a good idea.

▶ CHECKING YOUR ALIGNMENT

Once you are in Salamba Sarvangasana, adjust your alignment as described in this section to bring lightness and balance to your pose. First, check the balance between your right and left sides; then adjust the balance between your front body and back body; and finally, observe how your lower body rests on your upper body.

Balancing Your Right and Left Sides. When you first come into Salamba Sarvangasana, look up at the median line of your body—the line that runs from the tip of your nose through the center of your sternum and navel, and continues through the line of your inner legs. If this line is perpendicular, you are evenly balanced on your right and left shoulders. If the median line veers to one side or the other, your shoulders are imbalanced and the weight of your body falls more heavily on one side of your neck (Figure 1.7).

Are Your Shoulders Aligned with Your Blanket? If you discover an imbalance between your right and left shoulders in Salamba Sarvangasana, check that your shoulders are aligned evenly with the edge of your blanket.

First, lower your legs and come into Halasana (Figure 3.17). Then bring your fingertips to your shoulders, and measure the distance between the edge of your blanket and your right and left shoulders. If you have pulled one shoulder farther onto your blanket, adjust your shoulders so that they are equidistant from the edge of the blanket. (As a general rule, if you have one shoulder that is more flexible than the other, you may tend to pull that shoulder farther onto the blanket and strain that side of your neck.)

When you have adjusted your shoulders, place your hands flat on your back, raise your legs, and return to Salamba Sarvangasana. Once again, check the median line of your front body. Now that

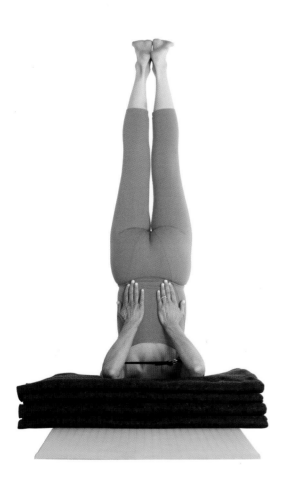

1.6
Salamba Sarvangasana,
Hands on Back
(back view)

your shoulders are properly aligned with the edge of your blanket, has the balance between your right and left sides improved?

Shoulder Imbalances. Stiffness or discomfort on one side of your neck is another indication that the weight of your body is distributed unevenly between your right and left shoulders. If the right side of your neck feels stiff or if your rib cage shifts to the right, your right shoulder blade does not lift away from the floor as much as your left, and your right elbow probably slides out to the side. To adjust your pose, firm the muscles at the back of your right armpit, press your right elbow down, and lift your right shoulder blade away from the floor. As you lift your right shoulder blade, your rib cage and pelvis should move closer to the center. (If your rib cage and pelvis shift to the left, make these adjustments on your left side.)

Using a Lift Under One Elbow. If you are unable to make the adjustment in the previous paragraph, place a folded mat or other support under your right elbow. This support will give you extra leverage as you press your elbow down. Continue to work with the lift under your elbow for a week or two, and then try once again to make the adjustment without this extra support. (If your rib cage and pelvis shift to the left, place the support under your left elbow.) Unless you have a pronounced scoliosis, eventually you will be able to bring your torso back into alignment without a lift under the elbow.

1.7
Salamba Sarvangasana (front view)

1.8
Salamba Sarvangasana (side view)

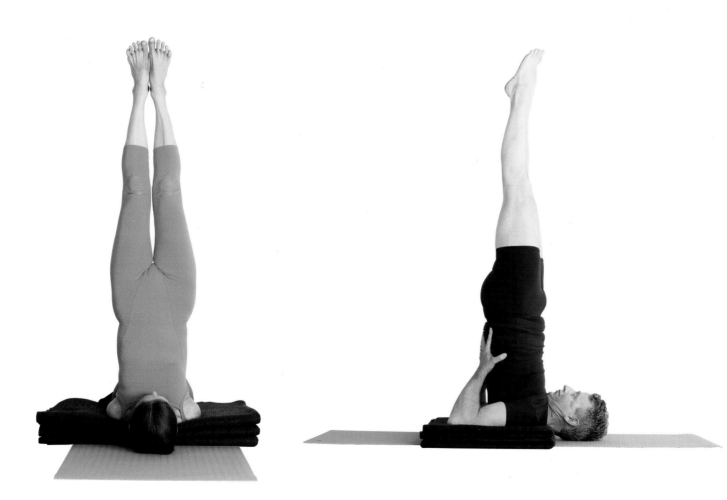

Adjusting Your Kidneys. Place your hands flat on your back with your palms broad and your fingers pointing toward your waist. Let your lower rib cage rest against your hands, and feel whether your kidneys are lifting away from or dropping into your palms. (Your kidneys are toward the back of your body, close to your spine and your floating ribs.) Then lift your kidneys away from your palms. If you have a shoulder imbalance, one kidney may be lifting and the other kidney dropping. Lift your kidneys evenly to balance your right and left sides. (For more information about the kidneys, see Chapter 5.)

Lifting Your Legs Evenly. Even if your shoulders are properly balanced, your pelvis and lumbar spine might be rotated. In this case, the median line of your torso will be centered, but the line of your inner legs will tilt to one side or the other: one leg is lifting and the other leg dropping. To lift your legs evenly, create maximum space between your thighbone and your pubic bone on each side. Lift your left thighbone away from the left side of your pubic bone, and your right thighbone away from the right side of your pubic bone. This adjustment should bring your pelvis and legs into better alignment.

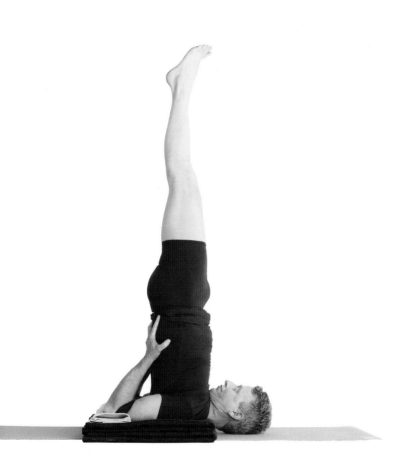

1.9
Salamba Sarvangasana, Lift Under the Elbows

Balancing Your Front Body and Back Body. Ideally, in Salamba Sarvangasana, the weight of your body should be evenly distributed between your elbows and your shoulders, so that you are balanced between your front body and back body. If your weight falls onto your shoulders and your elbows lift away from your blanket, you are pushing onto the front of your rib cage and may feel pressure on your neck. If your weight falls onto your elbows and your outer shoulders come away from your blanket, you are resting on your upper back, not lifting onto the ridge of your shoulders (Figure 1.8).

Weight on Shoulders, Not on Elbows. If your weight comes onto your shoulders and your elbows lift away from your blanket, you are either very flexible or using blankets that are too high. In either case, rest your rib cage on your hands and lean back onto your elbows, so that your upper arms bear the weight of the pose, rather than your shoulders and neck. If there is still a gap between your elbows and your blanket, place a folded nonskid mat under your elbows to provide support (Figure 1.9).

Do Not Push with Your Hands. If you are very flexible or using high blankets, be careful how you work with your hands to adjust your rib cage. Do not push your lower rib cage forward with your hands. This action forces your legs and pelvis forward so that they are no longer vertically aligned with your shoulders, and puts tremendous pressure on your neck. Instead of pushing your rib cage forward with your hands, lift your rib cage away from your hands. When you adjust in this way, your legs and pelvis will lift up and back, in line with your shoulders.

Weight on Elbows, Not on Shoulders. If your weight falls more heavily on your elbows than on your shoulders, increase the height of your support to three or four blankets. If you already use three or four blankets, put a folded nonskid mat under your elbows to give them an additional lift. Place the mat so that it supports the tips of your elbows only, not the middle of your upper arms.

If this additional support does not substantially improve your pose, your shoulders and upper back may not be ready for Salmaba Sarvangasana. In this case, practice Sarvangasana with a Chair (Figure 1.15) or Salamba Sarvangasana with Feet on the Wall (Figure 1.16) until you are able to lift higher onto your shoulders.

Checking the Median Line of Your Side Rib Cage. Ideally, in Salamba Sarvangasana your upper arms form a right angle with the sides of your rib cage to give maximum support. Your upper arms are then parallel to the floor, and the median line of your side rib cage is perpendicular to the floor.

To check the angle between your upper arms and the sides of your rib cage, you will need the help of a teacher or friend. If the angle is less than 90 degrees, you need a folded mat under your elbows so that you can press your elbows down. (See "Weight on Shoulders, Not on Elbows.") If the angle is greater than 90 degrees, you need a folded mat under your elbows to lift your elbows up. (See "Weight on Elbows, Not on Shoulders.") In either case, the folded mat should be just thick enough to bring your upper arms parallel to the floor.

Balancing Your Upper Body and Lower Body. In balancing your upper body and lower body, first check that your legs and pelvis are vertically aligned and then allow your spine to balance internally (Figure 1.10).

Are Your Legs Vertical? Once you have adjusted your upper body, check the position of your legs and pelvis by glancing upward. If your legs are not balanced directly over your pelvis, are they tilted forward or arching back?

If you are unsure about the alignment of your legs and pelvis, ask a teacher or friend to check your pose by looking at you from the side. When your legs and pelvis are properly balanced on your spine and rib cage, all your major joints are stacked vertically—ankles, knees, hip joints, and shoulder joints.

Legs Tilting Forward, Pelvis Dropping Back. If your legs are tilted forward but your pelvis drops back, move your perineum forward from your tailbone, roll your pubic bone toward your legs, and lengthen your front thighs toward your knees. Then firm the core of your buttocks, and lengthen your hamstrings toward the back of your knees until your legs are balanced vertically over your pelvis.

Legs Arching Back, Pelvis Pressing Forward. If your legs are arching back but your pelvis is pressing forward, you may be gripping your buttock muscles and pushing

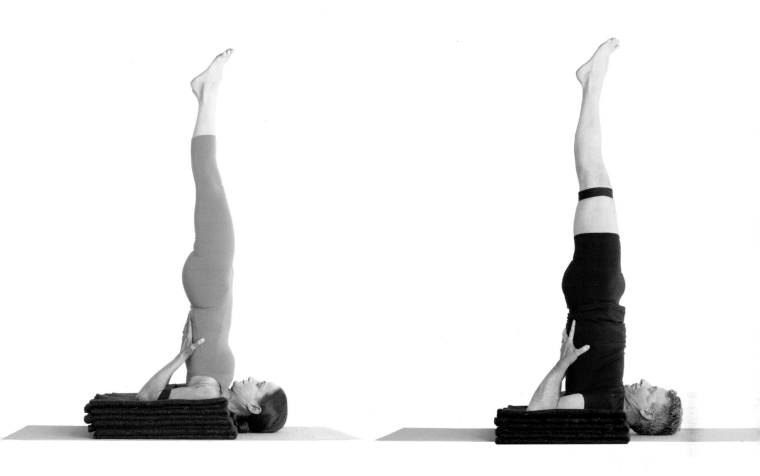

1.10
Salamba Sarvangasana

1.11
Salamba Sarvangasana with a Strap on the Thighs

your rib cage. In this case, let your rib cage rest back onto your hands, relax your buttocks, and draw your groins back into your body. Then firm your quadriceps and lengthen your hamstrings away from the core of your buttocks. Feel that your legs are supported evenly by your groins and quadriceps at the front of your body, and by your buttocks and hamstrings at the back of your body.

For Aching Backs and Sinking Legs. If you feel discomfort in your lower back in Salamba Sarvanagasana, or your legs feel heavy and lethargic, tie a strap above your knees to help lift your legs and take weight off your lower back.

Tie the strap snugly around your lower thighs, about 3 or 4 inches above your knees, so that your knees are lightly touching. (Do not tie the strap so tightly that you cannot lengthen your legs.) Once you are in Salamba Sarvangasana with a Strap on the Thighs (Figure 1.11), press your legs out against the strap, and lift your inner legs away from your inner groins. When you activate your legs in this way, your pose will feel much lighter.

Balancing Your Spine. Balancing your upper body and lower body in Salamba Sarvangasana comes ultimately from balancing your spine. Once you have adjusted your legs and pelvis as already described, draw your attention inward to your sacrum and spine. First lift your legs and let them balance on your sacrum. At the same time, adjust your pelvis so that your sacrum balances on your lumbar spine. Then bring your lumbar spine into balance with your thoracic spine. If you overwork your thoracic spine, allow it to relax and balance on your cervical spine. Finally, let your cervical spine lengthen toward the crown of your head to balance your neck and the base of your skull. At each stage, relinquish control of your outer body, so that your inner body can guide you to the place of lightness and balance in the pose. Let your effort be effortless!

▶
BEFORE SALAMBA SARVANGASANA CAUTIONS AND CONSIDERATIONS

This section contains cautions about practicing Salamba Sarvangasana and suggestions for alternative poses.

▶ Do not practice Salamba Sarvangasana during menstruation. If you attend a yoga class at this time, practice a reclining or restorative pose when the rest of the class is in Salamba Sarvangasana.

▶ If you are suffering from a stress-related headache or migraine, practice Viparita Karani (Figure 1.14) in place of Salamba Sarvangasana. If you have tension or tightness at the base of your skull, practice Savasana with a Neck Roll (Figure 1.12) for 5 minutes before Viparita Karani.

▶ If you have high blood pressure, practice Viparita Karani instead of Salamba Sarvangasana.

▶ If you are recovering from an illness, feel deeply fatigued, or simply need to replenish your energy, practice Viparita Karani in place of Salamba Sarvangasana.

▶ If you have asthma or acute sinus problems, practice Savasana with a Neck Roll for 5 minutes to relieve the tension at the base of your skull, followed by Viparita Karani for another 5 to 10 minutes, instead of Salamba Sarvangasana.

▶ If you are recovering from a neck injury, such as whiplash, start by practicing Savasana with a Neck Roll instead of Salamba Sarvangasana. When your neck feels less vulnerable, try Viparita Karani or Setu Bandhasana with a Roll under C7 (Figure 1.13).

▶ For lower back pain, practice Viparita Karani with your pelvis on the floor, not on a bolster, and your legs up the wall. If you experience lower back pain in Salamba Sarvangasana only, try practicing with a strap around your thighs, as described earlier in "For Aching Backs and Sinking Legs."

▶ If you have a pronounced scoliosis, practice Viparita Karani or Sarvangasana with a Chair (Figure 1.15) instead of Salamba Sarvangasana, and seek the guidance of an experienced yoga teacher.

▶ If you have any other health concerns, please consult a qualified yoga teacher or your health care professional before practicing Salamba Sarvangasana.

▶ ADVICE FOR BEGINNERS

If you have not practiced Salamba Sarvangasana before, I recommend that you seek the help of a qualified yoga teacher. Even if you have a yoga teacher, read the section "Cautions and Considerations" very carefully. If any health condition mentioned there applies to you, practice the alternative poses as suggested.

If you are ready to begin Salamba Sarvangasana, take the first ten days to become familiar with the main alternatives before attempting the full pose. Start by practicing Viparita Karani (Figure 1.14) and determine the best way to prop yourself in the pose so that you feel utterly comfortable. You will be grateful to return to Viparita Karani on days when you are fatigued or recovering from illness.

Then move on to Sarvangasana with a Chair (Figure 1.15) for another few days, until you feel confident that you can navigate into and out of the pose with ease. Make a note in your practice journal of how you arranged your props for this variation. Observe how Sarvangasana with a Chair stimulates your energy and opens your chest without exertion.

When you can lift the sides of your rib cage to a vertical position in Sarvangasana with a Chair, you can begin to practice Salamba Sarvangasana with Feet on the Wall (Figure 1.16), unless you have problems with your neck or shoulders. In Salamba Sarvangasana with Feet on the Wall, first, adjust your upper back with your feet on the wall; then maintain the lift of your rib cage as you lift first one leg, and then the other, away from the wall. When you can bring both legs away from the wall without losing the lift of your upper back, you are ready to practice Salamba Sarvangasana away from the wall on a regular basis.

▶ VARIATIONS AND ALTERNATIVES

SAVASANA WITH A NECK ROLL
RELAXATION POSE VARIATION

PROPS
- 1 nonskid mat
- 2 blankets
- 1 rolled mat
- 1 facecloth

OPTIONAL PROP
- 1 hand towel

1.12
Savasana
with a Neck Roll

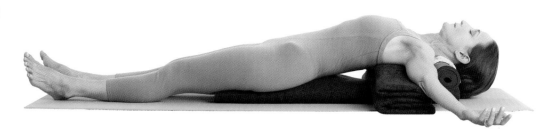

Savasana with a Neck Roll (Figure 1.12) is generally beneficial for those with neck problems or a reversed cervical curve because it restores and supports the natural curve of the neck. This variation also helps those who suffer from headaches, asthma, or sinus problems by releasing tension in the muscles at the base of the skull, which is often associated with these conditions.

For Savasana with a Neck Roll, you will need a nonskid mat to lie on, two standard folded blankets, another tightly rolled mat to support your neck, and a facecloth. Spread your first mat on the floor. Then fold one of your blankets in half lengthwise, and place it lengthwise on the mat. Fold the second blanket in thirds lengthwise, and place it crosswise on the first blanket, 4 or 5 inches from the top edge of the blanket. Balance your tightly rolled mat across the top edge of the first blanket, and cover the center of it with a facecloth so that the skin of your neck does not stick to the mat.

Now lie on your back with your pelvis resting on one end of the lengthwise blanket, your shoulder blades flat on the crosswise blanket, and the rolled mat directly underneath the middle of your neck, supporting the curve of your neck and the base of your skull. (If the rolled mat feels too harsh on your neck, use a hand towel instead. Fold the hand towel in half lengthwise, and roll it firmly from the narrow end, so that it is approximately 3 to 4 inches in diameter.)

In Savasana with a Neck Roll, extend your legs and then let them relax. Bend your elbows and rest your upper arms on the top edge of the crosswise blanket. Let your hands rest on the floor in line with your ears. Adjust the placement of your roll at the base of your skull so that your head hangs freely and your neck feels supported. When the roll is in place, close your eyes, broaden your forehead, and relax the base of your skull. The weight of your head should provide gentle traction for your cervical spine.

Remain in this position for 3 to 5 minutes. To come out, first bend your knees and place your feet flat on the floor, and then use your hands to lift your head and turn onto your right side. Press your hands into the floor to come to a sitting position.

Practice Notes. If you suffer from asthma or sinusitis, take a few moments to observe the effects of this pose. Do your sinuses feel clearer and wider? As you continue with your practice, notice after each pose how your sinuses are affected. Which poses tend to clear your sinuses, and which poses clog them? How is your breathing affected?

SETU BANDHASANA WITH A ROLL UNDER C7
BRIDGE POSE VARIATION

PROPS
- 1 nonskid mat
- 1 blanket
- 1 or 2 blocks
- 1 facecloth

OPTIONAL PROP
- 1 nonskid mat remnant

Setu Bandhasana with a Roll Under C7 (Figure 1.13) is recommended as an alternative to Salamba Sarvangasana (Figure 1.1) if you cannot put weight on your neck because of a reversed cervical curve or injury, such as whiplash. By supporting C7 and the upper thoracic vertebrae, the roll takes the weight off your neck, and allows you to relax your shoulders and lengthen your cervical spine.

For Setu Bandhasana with a Roll Under C7, you will need a nonskid mat, a folded blanket, one or two blocks, and a small, firm roll about 6 inches long and 2 inches in diameter. To make the roll, fold a facecloth in half lengthwise, and roll it tightly from the narrow end. (If you have the remnants of a nonskid mat available, cut a strip about 6 inches wide to make your roll. This material is firm and resilient, and gives better support. Secure the roll with rubber bands at each end.)

Fold a standard folded blanket in half lengthwise, and place it crosswise on your nonskid mat. Then lie with your shoulders at the folded edge of the blanket, and put the roll lengthwise under your C7 and T1–T3 (upper thoracic vertebrae). Extend your arms by your sides with your palms facing down and broaden your shoulders. Bend your knees, place your feet flat on the floor in line with your sitting bones, and lift your pelvis. Position a block, vertically on end, under your lower sacrum and tailbone to support your pelvis. (If you are tall or more flexible, use two blocks instead of one. Place the first block flat on the floor, and stack the second block on its end.)

CAUTION

Setu Bandhasana with a Roll Under C7 may not be helpful if you have an injury or misalignment in the area of C7 or the upper thoracic vertebrae. In any case, do not practice this variation if you experience pain or discomfort.

1.13
Setu Bandhasana with a Roll Under C7

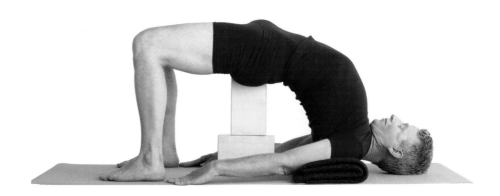

In Setu Bandhasana with a Roll Under C7, let your C7 and upper thoracic vertebrae sink into the roll as you lengthen the base of your skull away from your neck. (If the roll is not centered under your spine, or is not the right height, adjust the position or shape of your roll.) Then direct your breath into your upper rib cage, and let your shoulders relax toward the floor.

Maintain this position for 3 to 5 minutes. Lengthen the back of your upper arms toward your elbows, keep your shoulders wide, and lift your shoulder blades away from the floor without gripping your upper thoracic spine. Repeat this adjustment several times to learn this essential movement. To come out of the pose, lift your pelvis, remove the block, and rest your sacrum on the floor with your knees together.

Practice Notes. Remember to place the block under your *lower* sacrum and tailbone. If you place the block higher on your sacrum, you tend to flatten your lower back and put pressure on your sacroiliac joints. If you feel discomfort in your lower back no matter where the block is placed, practice this variation without blocks.

VIPARITA KARANI
SUPPORTED SHOULDERSTAND

PROPS
- 1 nonskid mat
- 1 or 2 blankets
- 1 bolster
- 1 strap
- 1 wall

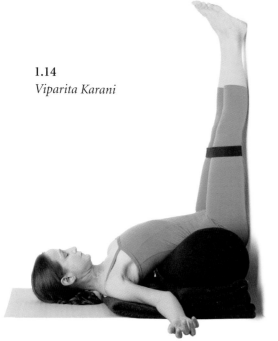

1.14
Viparita Karani

Viparita Karani (Figure 1.14) restores and replenishes energy more readily than any other pose, and is therefore beneficial when you are feeling fatigued or recovering from illness. Therapeutically, Viparita Karani lowers blood pressure, moderates breathing, and reduces tension in the body. If you have high blood pressure, suffer from asthma or other respiratory ailments, or experience migraines or stress-related headaches, Viparita Karani is an essential pose for you. If you have a chronic neck problem or very tight shoulders, Viparita Karani is a helpful alternative to Salamba Sarvangasana (Figure 1.1).

For Viparita Karani, use one blanket if you are shorter and two if you are taller. Lay your nonskid mat so that the short end is at the base of a wall. Fold your standard folded blankets in half lengthwise, and place them on the nonskid mat so that they are parallel with the wall, and 2 or 3 inches away from the wall. Place your bolster on top of the blankets.

Now sit at one end of the bolster with the left side of your body close to the wall. Tie the strap around your thighs just above your knees to hold your legs together. Then place your hands on the floor, turn your pelvis so that your sacrum rests firmly on the bolster, and extend your legs up the wall. Lower your head and shoulders to the floor, draw your shoulder blades away from your head, and place your arms out to the side. Close your eyes softly, and release the base of your skull away from the back of your neck.

Remain in this position for 5 to 10 minutes. With each inhalation, direct your breath toward your upper thoracic spine. With each exhalation, relax your shoulder blades. When you are ready to come out of the pose, bend your knees and remove the strap. Then slide off the bolster, and turn onto your right side. Lie in this position for a few breaths and then sit up.

Practice Notes. Ideally, the curve of your bolster should fit the curve of your lower back, giving support to your sacrum and floating ribs. If your lower back does not feel fully supported, your bolster may be too close to the wall. In this case, bend your knees and place your feet flat on the wall. Lift your pelvis and move your bolster and blankets a couple of inches farther away from the wall. Then rest your pelvis on the bolster once again, and extend your legs up the wall. When your bolster is positioned correctly, your tailbone and sitting bones are slightly lower than the top edge of your sacrum.

SARVANGASANA WITH A CHAIR
SHOULDERSTAND VARIATION

PROPS

- 1 chair
- 1 nonskid mat
- 2 or 3 blankets
- 1 folded nonskid mat

OPTIONAL PROPS

- 1 or 2 blankets
- 1 strap

In Sarvangasana with a Chair (Figure 1.15), your rib cage is arched, as in Setu Bandhasana with a Roll Under C7 (Figure 1.13), while your sacrum rests on the seat of the chair with your legs lifted vertically, as in full Salamba Sarvangasana (Figure 1.1).

This variation is helpful in a number of different circumstances. For example, if you have tight shoulders or a rounded upper back, Sarvangasana with a Chair helps you to open your chest and lift onto your shoulders. Or if you are recovering from a neck injury or have a pronounced scoliosis, the support of the chair keeps the weight of your legs and lower body from bearing down on your neck. Finally, if you are fatigued or recuperating from an illness, Sarvangasana with a Chair is more energizing and less demanding than full Salamba Sarvangasana.

Spread a nonskid mat lengthwise in front of your chair. Then stack two or three standard folded blankets, folded in half lengthwise, against the front of the chair, with the folded edges facing away from the chair. Fold another nonskid mat and place it on the seat of the chair so that it drapes over the front edge. This will provide some cushioning for your lower back.

Sit on the chair seat facing the back of the chair, and hang your lower legs over the backrest. Then lower your shoulders onto the blankets, and slide your pelvis toward the front edge of the chair. (You can rest your feet on the backrest of the chair, if you find it helpful.) With your head on the floor and your shoulders resting on the folded edge of the blankets, extend your arms between the legs of the chair, and take hold of the back legs of the chair. Lift your rib cage to come higher onto your shoulders. With your chest open and your sacrum resting on the chair seat, raise your legs toward the ceiling.

Hold this position for 3 to 10 minutes. Lengthen the back of your upper arms toward your elbows, keep your shoulders wide, and lift your shoulder blades away from the blankets. To come out of the pose, bend your knees, place your feet on the backrest of the chair, hold the front legs of the chair with your hands, and slide your shoulders and pelvis away from the chair. Then bring your knees into your chest and turn onto your side.

1.15
*Sarvangasana
with a Chair*

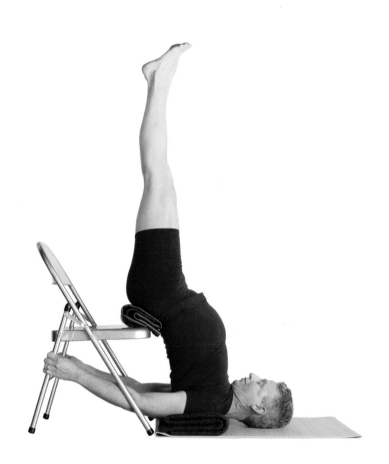

Practice Notes. The first few times you practice Sarvangasana with a Chair, you may need to adjust your props to suit your body proportions. If your torso is short, try adding another blanket or two to give additional height under your shoulders. If your torso is long, and the chair seat presses on your lumbar spine, place a folded blanket at the edge of the chair seat to give additional height and support for your sacrum. If you feel discomfort in your neck, try shifting your blankets either a little nearer to the chair or a little farther away, to give better support for your neck.

If your shoulders are wide, your arms might not fit easily between the legs of the chair. In this case, extend your arms outside the legs of the chair. If your arms are short, and you can't reach the back legs of the chair, tie a strap around the back legs of the chair and hold onto that. Be patient. It may take two or three attempts before you work out the optimum placement of props for this variation.

SALAMBA SARVANGASANA WITH FEET ON THE WALL
SHOULDERSTAND VARIATION

PROPS
- 1 nonskid mat
- 1 to 6 blankets
- 1 wall

OPTIONAL PROPS
- 1 bolster
- 1 strap

If you have difficulty lifting your rib cage in Salamba Sarvangasana (Figure 1.1), then Salamba Sarvangasana with Feet on the Wall (Figure 1.16) is a helpful variation. By resting your feet on the wall, you take the weight of the legs off the spine and can lift onto your shoulders more easily. This variation can also be practiced instead of Salamba Sarvangasana when you are fatigued or recovering from illness, and require a less strenuous pose.

Lay a nonskid mat with the short end at the base of a wall. Then place your blankets on the mat with the clean edges facing a wall, about 15 to 18 inches from the wall. If you are using three or more blankets, place a bolster lengthwise against your stack of blankets to support your pelvis and legs when lying down. Lie with your head pointing toward the wall and your shoulders at the folded edges of the blankets. Bend your knees and place your feet flat on the bolster in line with your sitting bones. With an inhalation, extend your arms by the sides of your torso, and press your shoulders into the blanket. With an exhalation, roll your pelvis away from the floor, and swing your legs overhead. Then extend your legs and rest your toes high on the wall.

In Salamba Sarvangasana with Feet on the Wall, walk your feet up the wall until your pelvis is aligned vertically over your shoulders. If you use a strap as recommended earlier in this chapter in "Using a Strap on Your Arms," widen your shoulders, press your arms out against the strap, and lift the back of your rib cage and your shoulder blades away from the floor. Repeat this adjustment two or three times. When your upper back is lifted as much as possible, bend your elbows and place your hands flat on your back with your fingers pointing toward your waist.

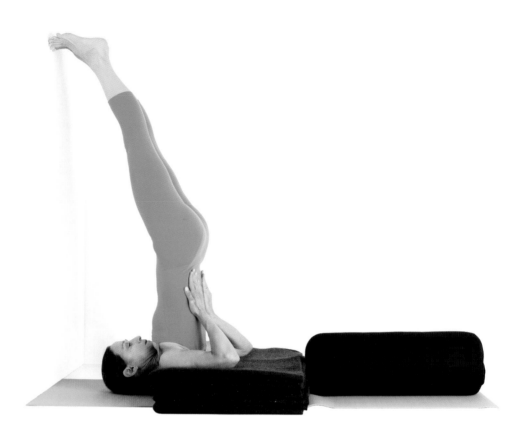

1.16
Salamba Sarvangasana
with Feet on the Wall

If you are not able to walk your feet high enough on the wall, move your blankets closer to the wall. However, if you feel any discomfort in your lower back, move your blankets farther away from the wall.

Maintain this position for 3 to 5 minutes. When you are ready, bend your knees, walk your feet down the wall, and slowly roll out of the pose. Rest with your feet flat on the bolster or floor.

Practice Notes. Once your pelvis is aligned directly over your shoulders, you can move to the next stage of the pose. Maintaining the lift of your rib cage, draw your right foot away from the wall, and lengthen your right leg toward the ceiling for several breaths. Then place your right foot back on the wall, bring your left foot away from the wall, and lengthen your left leg toward the ceiling for another few breaths.

Finally, keep your left leg extended, and bring your right leg away from the wall to meet it. You are now in Salamba Sarvangasana. If your rib cage collapses when you bring both legs away from the wall, return to Salamba Sarvangasana with Feet on the Wall. When you can keep both legs away from the wall for 1 to 2 minutes without losing the lift of your upper back, then you are ready to move away from the wall and practice Salamba Sarvangasana on a regular basis.

If you are practicing Salamba Sarvangasana with Feet on the Wall to recover from illness or fatigue, keep your feet on the wall throughout. Do not place your hands on your back. Instead, bend your elbows, rest your upper arms on the blanket in line with your shoulders, and place your hands on the floor in line with your ears. Relax your shoulders and release the base of your skull.

►
PRACTICE SUGGESTIONS

Timing Your Salamba Sarvangasana. When possible, include Salamba Sarvangasana (Figure 1.1) in your home yoga practice on a daily basis. Be consistent and practice the pose for the same amount of time each day. Use an electronic timer with a soft beep or a sports watch with a timing function to signal the end of the period.

Experienced practitioners can hold Salamba Sarvangasana for at least 10 minutes. However, if you are beginning a home practice, start with 1 or 2 minutes, and gradually add another 30 seconds to 1 minute throughout a period of weeks or months. Follow your practice of Salamba Sarvangasana with Halasana (Figure 3.17), lowering your legs to the floor or using a bolster, chair, or wall to support your feet if you have tight hamstrings. Hold Halasana for about one-third of the time you spent in Salamba Sarvangasana.

If your home practice is interrupted for more than a few days, you may need to reduce temporarily the amount of time you hold Salamba Sarvangasana once you resume your yoga routine. Do not immediately return to your previous level of practice, especially if you are recovering from illness, injury, or the effects of travel. Reduce your holding time by about one-third until you regain your strength and stamina.

More About Blankets. How many blankets should you use for Salamba Sarvangasana? Some teachers urge their students to use five or six blankets in Salamba Sarvangasana to protect their necks, while others, with equal conviction, reject the use of any blankets at all. I take the middle ground on this issue, because I have found higher blankets or lower blankets are appropriate for different students and different occasions.

I personally find great value in practicing Salamba Sarvangasana using both higher blankets (three or four) and lower blankets (one or two). I consider these blanket heights as two different variations. Salamba Sarvangasana with higher blankets allows me to lift my pelvis and legs more actively, and is anatomically easier on my body. Salamba Sarvangasana with lower blankets is more restful and, for me, triggers the deeper physiological benefits of the pose.

In my home practice, I begin with Salamba Sarvangasana on three or four blankets for the first 5 minutes to lift higher onto my shoulders and improve the alignment of my pelvis and legs. Then I practice Salamba Sarvangasana on one or two blankets for another 5 minutes, focusing on the movement of my breath and surrendering to the healing energy of the pose. Salamba Sarvangasana with higher blankets prepares me for practicing with lower blankets.

▶
SEQUENCING YOUR PRACTICE

In sequencing Salamba Sarvangasana (Figure 1.1) in your practice, take into account the time of day you intend to practice, your body type, and the other poses in your routine.

First, consider what poses to practice immediately before and immediately after Salamba Sarvangasana. If you are practicing Salamba Sirsasana (Figure 2.1), you can move directly into Salamba Sarvangasana. If you need more opening in your chest and shoulders, you can also include Adho Mukha Svanasana (Figure 3.4a), Setu Bandhasana with Blocks Under the Sacrum (Figure 8.20), or Bharadvajasana II (Figure 6.16) immediately before Salamba Sarvangasana.

Immediately after Salamba Sarvangasana, come into Halasana (Figure 3.17) for about one-third of the time you spent in Salamba Sarvangasana. If you feel discomfort in your lower back or rib cage, include a lying twist or seated twist to release your spine after Halasana. If your neck and shoulders feel tense, practice Anantasana with a Bolster (Figure 8.22) to release your cervical spine.

Then consider how Salamba Sarvangasana fits into the overall scheme of your practice. Following are some general guidelines for sequencing Salamba Sarvangasana in relation to different types of poses: inverted poses, standing poses, backbends, sitting twists, and sitting forward bends.

Inverted Poses. Practice Salamba Sarvangasana after other inverted poses, such as Adho Mukha Vrksasana at the Wall (Figure 3.11a), Pincha Mayurasana at the Wall (Figure 5.12), and Salamba Sirsasana (Figure 2.1). You can safely practice Salamba Sarvangasana without practicing Salamba Sirsasana, but if you practice Salamba Sirsasana, then Salamba Sarvangasana should follow later in your sequence. Salamba Sarvangasana is the ideal counterpose for Salamba Sirsasana: the latter pose tends to compress the curve of your neck, whereas the former pose helps to lengthen it.

Standing Poses. As a general rule, practice Salamba Sarvangasana after standing poses. Standing poses warm the body in preparation for inverted poses.

Backbends. Practice Salamba Sarvangasana after backbends, not before. Backbends can be overly stimulating to the nervous system, especially when practiced in the evening. Practicing Salamba Sarvangasana as a counterpose after a series of backbends helps to soothe the nerves, quiet the brain, and reduce agitation. If you suffer from insomnia after practicing backbends, end your practice sequence with Viparita Karani (Figure 1.14). If you prefer to end with full Salamba Sarvangasana, follow it with Halasana (Figure 3.17) with your legs supported by a chair or bench for at least 5 minutes.

Sitting Twists. Sitting twists are transition poses that help to balance and neutralize your spine. You can practice them beneficially either before or after Salamba Sarvangasana. When practiced before Salamba Sarvangasana, they create flexibility in your shoulders and cervical spine. When practiced after Salamba Sarvangasana, sitting twists function as counterposes by releasing tension and discomfort in your neck, thoracic spine, and lower back.

Sitting Forward Bends. Practice Salamba Sarvangasana before sitting forward bends, rather than after. Include variations, such as Ekapada Sarvangasana, in which one leg is lowered directly to the floor, and Parsvaikapada Sarvanagasana, in which one leg is lowered out to the side, to release your hip joints and gently stretch your hamstrings in preparation for sitting forward bends. Sitting forward bends calm your nervous system and pacify your mind, so Salamba Sarvangasana can feel heavy and dull if practiced afterward.

2 SALAMBA SIRSASANA

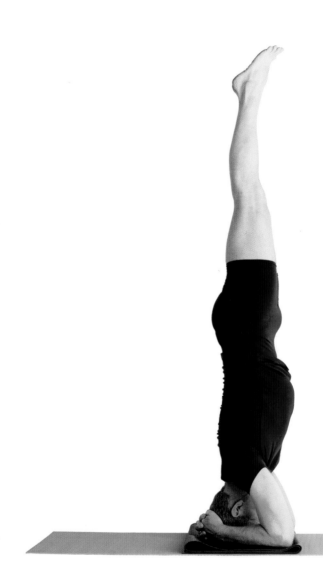

TRADITIONALLY, SALAMBA SARVANGASANA (Figure 1.1) has been regarded as the mother of all poses because of its nurturing quality, and Salamba Sirsasana (Figure 2.1) as the father of all poses because of its clarifying effect. Initially, Salamba Sirsasana is a challenging pose that requires strength in your arms and flexibility in your shoulders to avoid compression in your neck, as well as strength in your lower back and abdomen to support the weight of your legs. Ultimately, however, you will discover the place of inner balance in the pose, where your mind is clear and alert, your body calm and suspended, and your whole being poised between action and reflection.

CAUTION

If you have never practiced Salamba Sirsasana or you are unsure whether the pose is appropriate for you, please read "Cautions and Considerations" (p. 49) and "Advice for Beginners" (p. 50) before proceeding.

SALAMBA SIRSASANA
HEADSTAND

PROPS	OPTIONAL PROPS	
• 1 nonskid mat	• 1 blanket	• 1 strap
	• 1 facecloth or hand towel	• 1 tennis ball
	• 2 mats or blankets	• 1 nonskid mat remnant

ESTABLISHING YOUR FOUNDATION

For your comfort and ease in Salamba Sirsasana, use a folded blanket or mat as your foundation, so that your head and forearms are not in direct contact with the hard floor. Make sure the blanket is a firm one. If you use a fluffy blanket, your pose will feel unstable. Place your blanket on a nonskid mat to keep it from slipping.

If you prefer to use a folded nonskid mat, the same considerations apply. You need a firm, unwavering foundation under your forearms and head. If your nonskid mat is too thick and spongy, your pose will not feel secure.

Evaluating the Length of Your Arms. You may require additional props in Salamba Sirsasana, depending upon your body type and your proportions. In particular, the relationship between the length of your upper arms and the length of your head and neck is crucial. Here is a simple way to test this for yourself.

Sit in a kneeling position with your sitting bones resting on your heels, or at the edge of a folding chair if you are unable to kneel. Raise your arms overhead and interlock your fingers. Then bend your elbows and bring your forearms parallel to the ceiling.

facing page:
2.1
Salamba Sirsasana

Support Under Your Head. If your forearms are raised 1 or more inches above the crown of your head, then your upper arms are proportionally long in relation to your head and neck (Figure 2.2). In this case, your shoulders may feel compressed in Salamba Sirsasana because you have no room to lengthen your arms. To remedy this situation, place an extra support under your head to give you additional height. You can use a folded facecloth, a folded hand towel, or even a folded blanket. The support can range from ½ inch to 3 inches in thickness, depending on the disparity between the length of your upper arms and the length of your head and neck. Experiment with different thicknesses to determine which height works best for you. If your lift is too high, your head and neck will feel jammed, so when in doubt, use less rather than more.

2.2
Support Under the Head

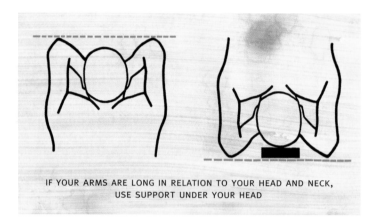

IF YOUR ARMS ARE LONG IN RELATION TO YOUR HEAD AND NECK,
USE SUPPORT UNDER YOUR HEAD

Support Under Your Forearms. If the crown of your head rises above the level of your forearms, then your head and neck are relatively long in comparison with your upper arms (Figure 2.3). In this case (which, by the way, is much less common), your neck may feel compressed in Salamba Sirsasana because your head—rather than your arms—bears most of the weight. To alleviate this situation, place additional support under your forearms to give extra space for your head and neck to lengthen. Use two nonskid mats folded into strips that measure ½ to 1 inch thick, or even higher if that feels comfortable. (You can use two folded blankets, but make sure the blankets are the same size and thickness.) Arrange your folded strips in a V shape on your foundation blanket, so that your forearms are raised and your head fits into the space between the folded strips.

2.3
Support Under the Forearms

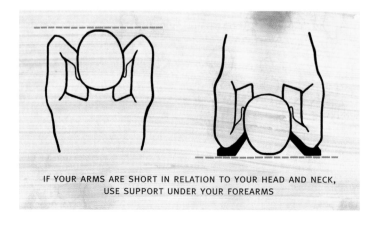

IF YOUR ARMS ARE SHORT IN RELATION TO YOUR HEAD AND NECK,
USE SUPPORT UNDER YOUR FOREARMS

Position Your Elbows. Kneel in front of your folded blanket, and place the tips of your elbows directly in line with the center of your shoulder joints, so that your upper arms are parallel to each other, and your weight rests evenly on your inner and outer elbows. Make sure that your elbows are equidistant from the front edge of the blanket.

If your elbows are too far apart, then your weight falls onto your inner elbows, and your inner arms lengthen more than your outer arms (Figure 2.4). If your elbows are too close together, then your weight falls onto your outer elbows, and your outer arms lengthen more than your inner arms. Distribute your weight evenly on your inner and outer elbows, so that your inner and outer arms give equal support.

2.4
Aligning Your Elbows
and Shoulder Joints

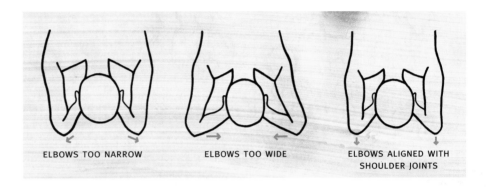

ELBOWS TOO NARROW   ELBOWS TOO WIDE   ELBOWS ALIGNED WITH
SHOULDER JOINTS

Interlock Your Fingers. When you interlock your hands, bring the roots of your fingers firmly together, so that the cup of your hands is strong and stable. Do not leave any space between the webs of your fingers and the opposite hand. Cross one thumb lightly over the other, so that the bottom knuckles of your thumbs are evenly aligned. Check that your wrists are equidistant from the edge of your blanket.

Change the Interlock. Remember to change the interlock of your fingers on a regular basis to avoid strengthening one side of your body at the expense of the other. For example, if you practice Salamba Sirsasana six days a week, you can cross your left hand over your right hand on Mondays, Wednesdays, and Fridays, and your right hand over your left hand on Tuesdays, Thursdays, and Saturdays.

I prefer to change the interlock of my fingers on a daily basis. I practice Salamba Sirsasana for 3 to 5 minutes with my left hand crossed over my right, and repeat the pose for another 3 to 5 minutes with my right hand crossed over my left. When I began practicing this way, my first Salamba Sirsasana felt stable and secure, but my second one was shaky and uncoordinated. With time and practice, my second pose now feels as strong and integrated as my first.

Place Your Outer Hands. When you place your outer hands on your blanket with your fingers interlocked, the cross of your little fingers may feel awkward and uncomfortable. Try this alternative: place the little finger of one hand inside the little finger of the other hand, so that the outer edges of both little fingers are in contact with your blanket. For me, this variation gives greater ease and stability.

Activate Your Hands Without Gripping. When you squeeze your fingers together and grip your hands in Salamba Sirsasana, the muscles at the sides of your neck automatically tighten. When you let your hands relax completely, they give no support in the pose. Here is a way to activate your hands without gripping. When your hands are interlocked, relax and lengthen your fingers, and then gently press your fingertips against the back of your hands and widen your palms.

Lengthen Your Outer Wrists. To bring your outer wrists into firm contact with your blanket, turn the mounds of your thumbs toward your inner wrists, and lengthen your outer hands away from your outer wrists. Then lengthen your forearms from your wrists to your elbows, so that your forearm bones press evenly into your blanket or mat.

Feel the Edges of Your Forearm Bones. If you have strong, muscular forearms, the sheer bulk of your forearm muscles may interfere with the placement of your forearm bones. Before positioning your forearms on your blanket for Salamba Sirsasana, press the fingertips of your left hand along the inner edge of your right forearm bone, and lift your inner forearm muscle away from the bone. Then repeat on the other side. As you place your forearms on the blanket, let your inner forearms soften, so that you rest directly on your forearm bones.

In Salamba Sirsasana, check that your forearm bones are in firm contact with your blanket all the way from your outer wrists to your elbows. Relax your inner forearm muscles, and lift your outer forearm muscles away from the floor, so that your forearm bones can sink deeper into your blanket.

Lower Your Head. Once you have placed your elbows, forearms, and hands on the blanket, widen your shoulder blades and lift your shoulders, but let your head and neck hang freely, so that the crown of your head directly faces the floor. Then slowly release your shoulders and lower your head, letting gravity be your guide.

When the crown of your head rests squarely on your blanket, adjust the cup of your hands to support the back of your head. Bring your hands to your head, not your head to your hands! (For more details about adjusting the cup of your hands, see "Checking the Placement of Your Head," later in this chapter.)

The Crown of Your Head. To maintain the natural curve of your neck in Salamba Sirsasana, the weight should be centered on the crown of your head. If your weight is too far forward, your cervical spine will be overarched. If your weight is too far back, your cervical spine will be flattened.

Test this for yourself by standing in Tadasana (Figure 3.3) and placing the palm of one hand on the crown of your head (Figure 2.5). First, lift the front edge of the crown of your head higher than the back edge. Observe how your chin lifts, your head drops back, and your cervical spine feels more compressed. Next, lift the back edge of the crown of your head higher than the front edge. Feel how your chin tucks, your head comes forward, and your cervical spine flattens. Finally, lift the front edge and the back edge of the crown of your head evenly into the palm of your hand, and feel how your whole spine lengthens. This neutral position is the best way to protect your neck in this physically demanding pose.

Soften Your Gaze. In Salamba Sirsasana, rest your eyes on your lower lids and

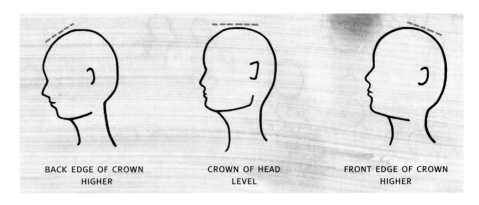

BACK EDGE OF CROWN
HIGHER

CROWN OF HEAD
LEVEL

FRONT EDGE OF CROWN
HIGHER

soften your gaze, looking directly ahead, not down at the floor. If you habitually stare at the floor in Salamba Sirsasana to give yourself a sense of security, you may be creating tension in your eyes and at the base of your skull, and you may be shifting your weight forward on your head.

Raising Your Legs. Once you have placed the crown of your head on the blanket between your forearms, turn your toes under, lift your knees, and straighten your legs. Widen your shoulder blades and press your elbows into the blanket to stabilize your rib cage as you walk your feet in 2 or 3 inches. Then pause, draw your lower abdomen toward your sacrum to lift your pelvis higher, and walk your feet in another couple of inches.

Coming Up with Bent Knees. If you are a beginner with Salamba Sirsasana, lift your right knee into your chest, and bring your right heel toward your right sitting bone. Then push your left toes into the floor, draw your left knee into your chest, and bring your left foot to meet your right foot. Keep your heels close to your sitting bones, raise your knees toward the ceiling, and straighten your legs. You are now in Salamba Sirsasana.

When you have developed strength in your lower abdomen, you will be able to lift both knees into your chest simultaneously. (See "Coming Down with Bent Knees" and "Coming Down with Straight Legs," later in this chapter, for suggestions on how to develop strength and coordination for this movement.)

Coming Up with Straight Legs. Once you can draw both knees into your chest simultaneously, you can try coming into Salamba Sirsasana with your legs straight. As you walk your feet toward your elbows and lift your lower abdomen toward your sacrum, observe what happens to your feet and toes. If your toes feel lighter on the floor and your legs begin to levitate, you are ready to come up with your legs straight. Wait for your body to give you the signal!

Practice coming down with straight legs before you attempt to come up with straight legs. Once you are adept at coming down quietly and smoothly with straight legs, without making a thumping sound as your feet touch the floor, you can safely consider coming up with straight legs. (See "Coming Down with Bent Knees" or "Coming Down with Straight Legs," later in this chapter.)

To protect your neck when coming into Salamba Sirsasana, stabilize your rib cage by widening your shoulder blades and pressing your elbows into the blanket as you walk your feet in. Let your rib cage and legs move toward each other: action and counteraction. Do not walk your feet in as far as possible: instead, walk your feet in the least amount necessary to come up with straight legs. When you walk your feet in as far as possible, you raise your legs by arching your back and contracting your paraspinal muscles. When you walk your feet in the least amount necesary, you raise your legs from the strength of your lower abdomen.

▶
CHECKING YOUR ALIGNMENT

2.6
Salamba Sirsasana

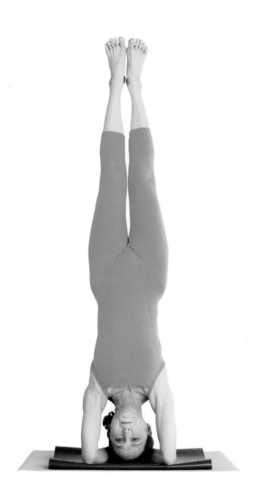

Once you are in Salamba Sirsasana, check your alignment, as described in the following sections, to protect your neck and enhance your balance. First, compare your right and left sides; next, adjust the balance between your front body and back body; and finally, observe how your lower body balances on your upper body.

Balancing Your Right and Left Sides. Many students experience an imbalance between their right and left sides in Salamba Sirsasana (Figure 2.6). The source of this imbalance is different for different people. The following sections help you to determine which areas of your body require your special attention in balancing your right and left sides.

Is Your Head Tilted to One Side? If your head is tilted to the right or left, one side of your neck is bearing more weight than the other. This can lead to stiffness or discomfort on the side where your neck is compressed. To adjust the tilt of your head, align your inner ears so that they are equidistant from the floor on your right side and left side, and parallel to the frontal plane of your body.

Does One Elbow Slide Out More Than the Other? If one elbow slides out more than the other, your arms do not support you evenly on your right and left sides. To adjust your arms, check that your weight is evenly distributed between your inner and outer elbows. On your stable side, observe how your weight falls equally on your inner and outer elbows. On the side where your arm slides out, notice how your weight falls more on your inner elbow. Press your wandering elbow toward the median line of the body, and stabilize your inner and outer elbows. (For more details about stabilizing your elbows, see Chapter 7.)

If your elbow continues to slide despite these adjustments, place a nonskid mat over your blanket so that your practice surface is less slippery or use a strap around your elbows to hold them in place. (Make sure the strap is not too tight.)

Are Your Collarbones Level? When your shoulder girdle is balanced in Salamba Sirsasana, your right and left collarbones are parallel with the frontal plane of your body (Figure 2.7). However, if the outer corner of one collarbone moves forward, but the other one falls back, then one of

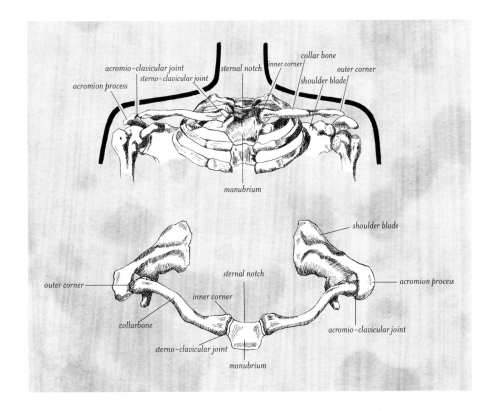

your shoulders is lifting and the other one is dropping, and your shoulder girdle is imbalanced.

To adjust your shoulders, focus on the side where the outer corner of your collarbone falls back. First, relax the acromio-clavicular joint, where the outer corner of your collarbone attaches onto your outer shoulder blade. (This joint may feel stuck.) Then gently lengthen your upper arm, and move the outer corner of your collarbone forward, until both collarbones are parallel to the frontal plane of your body. When your collarbones are level, press down with your elbows and lift your rib cage away from the outer corners of your collarbones; lift evenly on your right and left sides. (See Chapter 5 for more information about the collarbones.)

Lifting Your Legs Evenly. Even if your shoulders are properly balanced, your pelvis and lumbar spine may be rotated. In this case, one leg is lifting and the other leg dropping. To lift your legs evenly, create maximum space between your thighbone and your pubic bone on each side. Lift your left thighbone away from the left side of your pubic bone, and lift your right thighbone away from the right side of your pubic bone. This adjustment should bring your pelvis and legs into better alignment.

Balancing Your Front Body and Back Body. In balancing your front body and back body, first check that your head is positioned correctly, and then observe how your weight is distributed between your elbows and wrists (Figure 2.8).

Checking the Placement of Your Head. Ask a teacher or an experienced yoga practitioner to check the placement of your head in Salamba Sirsasana by standing to one side and looking at the relationship between your ears and your shoulder joints. If your ears are vertically aligned with your shoulder joints, then the crown of your head is correctly placed (Figure 2.9). If your ears are not directly under your shoulder joints, but nearer to your hands, then your head is placed too far back. If your ears are not in line with your shoulder joints, but nearer to your elbows, then your head is placed too far forward.

If a teacher or friend is unavailable, here are some cues to help you assess the position of your head. When you place your head too far back, you will feel that the weight of your body is transmitted through your jawbone, that is, in front of your ears. If you place your head too far forward, you will feel the weight of your body falling on the back of your skull, behind your ears. When the crown of your head is correctly placed, the weight of your body passes directly through the center of your ears.

Head Placed Too Far Back. When you place your head too far back in your hands, the top of your head rests closer to your forehead instead of on the crown of your head, and your cervical spine is overarched. In this case, the cup of your hands is too wide in relation to your head and neck.

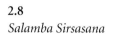

2.8
Salamba Sirsasana

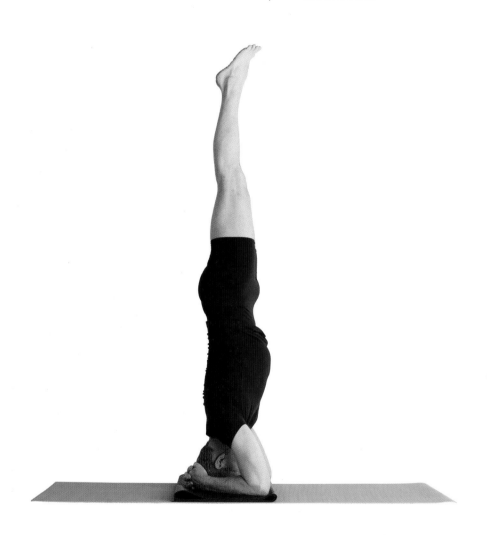

ing forward and your pelvis tilting back. If your inner anklebones are behind your sitting bones, then your legs are arching back and your pelvis pressing forward. When your inner anklebones are directly above your sitting bones, then your legs are vertically aligned.

If you are not sure about the alignment of your legs, ask a teacher or friend to look at your pose from the side. When your legs are vertical, the centers of your ankles, knees, and hip joints are vertically aligned with one another.

Legs Tilting Forward, Pelvis Tilting Back. If your legs are tilting forward and your pelvis is tilting back, then you are holding your legs from your groins and your quadriceps, and not engaging your buttocks or hamstrings. In this case, move your perineum forward from your tailbone, roll your pubic bone toward your thighs, and lengthen the fronts of your thighs toward your knees. At the same time, firm the core of your buttocks against your pelvis, and lengthen your hamstrings from the core of your buttocks to the back of your knees.

Legs Arching Back, Pelvis Pressing Forward. If your legs are arching back and your pelvis pressing forward, then you are probably gripping your buttocks and over-

2.11
Salamba Sirsasana

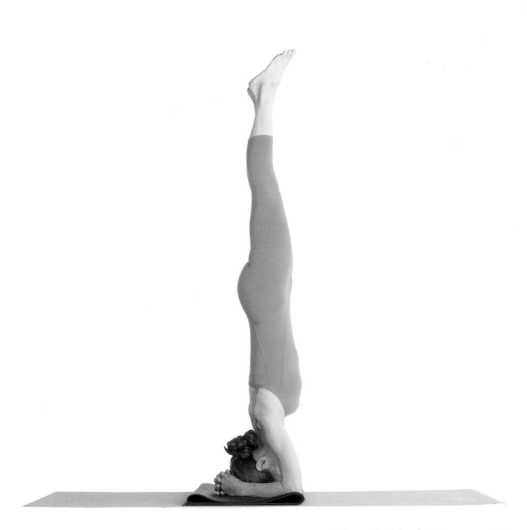

working the back of your body. In this case, move your groins back and firm your quadriceps. At the same time, relax the gripping action of your buttocks, and lengthen your hamstrings from the core of your buttocks to the back of your knees.

When you support your legs evenly from your groins and quadriceps at the front of the body, and your buttocks and hamstrings at the back of the body, your legs will naturally return to a vertical position.

Balancing the Spine. When your upper body is stable and your legs are vertically aligned, bring your awareness to the core of your body, and allow your spine to find its own place of balance. Let your legs rest on the platform of your sacrum. Let the curve of your lumbar spine balance on the curve of your thoracic spine. Let the curve of your thoracic spine balance on the curve of your cervical spine. Feel the weight on the crown of your head, and the lightness and length of your neck. Maintain this inward focus to strengthen and balance your spine.

If you are an experienced practitioner, be aware that overworking your arms can interfere with the balance and alignment of your spine. Ultimately, Salamba Sirsasana is a balancing pose, not a buttressing pose.

▶ COMING DOWN FROM SALAMBA SIRSASANA

If you practice Salamba Sirsasana at the Wall (Figure 2.14) or Salamba Sirsasana with Blocks at the Wall (Figure 2.16a), come down with your knees bent. Do not attempt to come down with your legs straight. If you practice Salamba Sirsasana near the Wall (Figure 2.15) or if you practice Salamba Sirsasana in the middle of the room, come down with your legs straight; however, do this only after you have mastered coming down with bent knees, using the strength of your lower abdomen, as described in the following section.

Coming Down with Bent Knees. If you practice Salamba Sirsasana at the Wall or Salamba Sirsasana near the Wall, bend your knees and slide your feet down the wall toward your pelvis. As your heels come closer to your sitting bones, press your elbows down firmly, roll your lower abdomen toward your sacrum, and bring your knees and thighs toward your rib cage. Maintain this position from the strength of your lower abdomen for several seconds. Once again, press your elbows down firmly, roll your lower abdomen toward your sacrum, and drop your feet to the floor. Rest in Adho Mukha Virasana (Child's Pose, Figure 3.11b) until your breathing returns to normal.

When you come down with bent knees, do you come down evenly with your right and left legs, or does one side lead the other? Is the movement smooth and sustained throughout, or do you lose control halfway through? Continue to practice coming down with bent knees until you can come down smoothly and evenly on a regular basis; then try coming down with straight legs.

Coming Down with Straight Legs. To come down with straight legs, first widen your collarbones and lift the sides of your rib cage away from your elbows to stabilize your upper body. Then release your inner groins, draw your lower abdomen toward your sacrum, and lengthen your inner hamstrings as you lower your legs. When your toes touch the floor, bend your knees and rest for several breaths in Adho Mukha Virasana.

Listen to Your Feet. If your feet hit the floor with a thump, you are probably arching your lower back and using your paraspinal muscles, rather than your abdominal muscles, to control the movement. In this case, practice Salamba Sirsasana coming up and down with bent knees to develop the strength and awareness of your lower abdomen in this pose. Once you have learned how to control the movement from the core of your abdomen, resume coming up and down with your legs straight.

▶
Before Salamba Sirsasana
Cautions and Considerations

This section has cautions about practicing Salamba Sirsasana (Figure 2.1) and suggestions for alternative poses.

▶ Do not practice Salamba Sirasana during menstruation. If you attend a yoga class at this time, practice a reclining or restorative pose while the rest of the class is in Salamba Sirsasana.

▶ If you are suffering from a stress-related headache or migraine, practice Prasarita Padottanasana (Figure 2.13b) in place of Salamba Sirsasana.

▶ If you have asthma or acute sinus problems, practice Savasana with a Neck Roll (Figure 1.12), as described in Chapter 1, for a few minutes to relieve tension at the base of your skull before you practice Salamba Sirsasana.

▶ If you have high blood pressure or heart problems, practice Adho Mukha Svanasana with Forehead Support (Figure 2.12) instead of Salamba Sirsasana.

▶ If you have lower back pain, practice Adho Mukha Svanasana with Forehead Support instead of Salamba Sirsasana.

▶ If you are recovering from an illness or feel deeply fatigued, practice Adho Mukha Svanasana with Forehead Support for a few minutes before Salamba Sirsasana. If you are feeling weak or shaky, practice Salamba Sirsasana at the Wall (Figure 2.14).

▶ If you are recovering from a neck injury, such as whiplash, start by practicing Prasarita Padottanasana instead of Salamba Sirsasana. When you feel ready to attempt Salamba Sirsasana, seek the advice of an experienced yoga teacher.

▶ If you have a scoliosis, practice Prasarita Padottanasana instead of Salamba Sirsasana. If you are eager to try Salamba Sirsasana, seek the guidance of an experienced teacher. With careful attention to the placement of props, you may safely practice Salamba Sirsasana with Blocks at the Wall (Figure 2.16a) if your scoliosis is mild or moderate.

▶ If you have a history of detached retina, do not practice Salamba Sirsasana without consulting an experienced yoga teacher.

▶ If you experience any discomfort in your neck or pressure in your eyes in any variation of Salamba Sirsasana, discontinue your practice of the pose for the time being, and seek the advice of your ongoing yoga teacher and your health care practitioner.

▶ If you have any other health concerns, consult an experienced yoga teacher or your health care professional before practicing Salamba Sirsasana.

▶
ADVICE FOR BEGINNERS

If you have not practiced Salamba Sirsasana (Figure 2.1) before, I recommend that you seek the help of an experienced teacher. In any case, read "Cautions and Considerations" carefully. If any of the health conditions mentioned there apply to you, practice the alternative poses that I recommend.

When you are ready to practice Salamba Sirsasana, begin by reading the instructions for Salamba Sirsasana in this chapter. In general, the instructions for freestanding Salamba Sirsasana apply to Salamba Sirsasana at the Wall (Figure 2.14) and Salamba Sirsasana near the Wall (Figure 2.15) as well. In particular, the section "Evaluating the Length of Your Arms" will help you determine whether you need additional support under your head or forearms.

Start by practicing Salamba Sirsasana at the Wall, at least for the first few days. When you can bring your legs away from the wall and your balance is steady, move to Salamba Sirsasana near the Wall. When you can balance in Salamba Sirsasana near the Wall for 1 or 2 minutes without using the support of the wall, try moving to the center of the room.

If you want to practice Salamba Sirsasana with Blocks at the Wall (Figure 2.16a), seek the advice of an experienced teacher, who can help you arrange the blocks appropriately and check your alignment.

ADHO MUKHA SVANASANA WITH FOREHEAD SUPPORT
DOWNWARD-FACING DOG POSE VARIATION

PROPS
- 1 nonskid mat
- 2 blocks

OPTIONAL PROP
- 1 wedge

Adho Mukha Svanasana with Forehead Support (Figure 2.12) is an excellent warm-up for Salamba Sirsasana (Figure 2.1), and an ideal alternative if you are not yet ready to place weight on your head. This preparation opens your shoulders, releases tension at the base of your skull, and relaxes your neck.

Kneel on a nonskid mat, and sit back on your heels. Stack two blocks on your mat about 10 inches in front of your knees. Set the first block flat and the second block on its side. Then come to a kneeling position, and place your hands on the mat in line with your shoulders. Turn your toes under, lift your pelvis, and straighten your legs so that your whole forehead rests comfortably on the blocks. You may need to adjust the position or height of your blocks. (If your heels don't touch the floor, use a wedge under your heels to support them.)

2.12
Adho Mukha Svanasana with Forehead Support

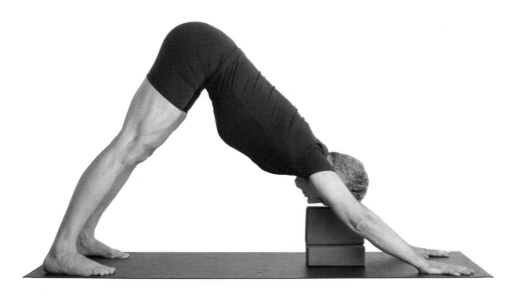

In Adho Mukha Svanasana with Forehead Support, relax your shoulders and widen your shoulder blades. Then broaden your palms, firm your inner elbows, and lengthen the sides of your chest. At the same time, draw your groins into your body, and bring your weight back onto your legs. Maintain this position for about 1 minute, breathing softly; then bend your knees and rest in Adho Mukha Virasana (Child's Pose, Figure 3.11b). If you are practicing this variation as an alternative to Salamba Sirsasana, repeat two or three times.

Practice Notes. If you have flexible shoulders, do not sink into your shoulder joints. If you feel your rib cage collapsing, walk your hands out a bit farther, and lengthen the sides of your rib cage away from your inner elbows. This adjustment will strengthen your arms, lift your rib cage, and create space in your shoulder joints.

PRASARITA PADOTTANASANA
WIDE-LEG STANDING FORWARD BEND

PROP	OPTIONAL PROP
• 1 nonskid mat	• 1 block
	• 1 blanket

2.13a
Prasarita Padottanasana, Phase 1

If you are unable to practice Salamba Sirsasana (Figure 2.1) because of a neck or shoulder injury, high blood pressure, or other contraindicated condition, Prasarita Padottanasana is an excellent alternative. The second phase of this pose (Figure 2.13b)

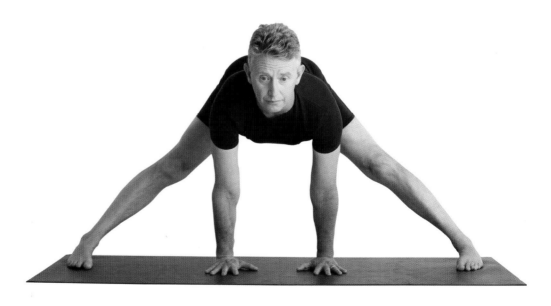

gives you many of the physiological benefits of an inverted pose without placing weight on your head or neck.

Stand in Tadasana (Figure 3.3) on a nonskid mat, and separate your legs 4 to 4½ feet apart with your feet parallel. Place your hands on your hips with your thumbs pressing the top edge of your sacrum. With an inhalation, lift the sides of your rib cage, and let your head drop back if it feels comfortable on your neck. With an exhalation, draw your groins up into your body and extend your torso forward until your spine is parallel to the floor. Then extend your arms and place your fingertips on the floor in line with your toes. (Use a block under your hands if you cannot reach the floor without rounding your back.)

Phase 1. In the first phase of Prasarita Padottanasana (Figure 2.13a), your spine is extended in a gentle backbend. Maintain this position for several breaths, firming your hamstrings and lifting the sides of your rib cage away from your inner elbows. Then, with an inhalation, draw your groins into your body, and lengthen your spine through the crown of your head. With an exhalation, bend your elbows and rest the crown of your head on the floor. (If the crown of your head does not touch the floor, use a block or folded blanket for support.) Move your hands back so that they are in line with your heels, your upper arms are parallel to each other, and your elbows form a right angle.

Phase 2. In the second phase of Prasarita Padottanasana (Figure 2.13b), your spine is gently rounded in a forward bend. Firm your hamstrings and lift your groins into your body to release your lumbar spine. Broaden your midsternum to relax your thoracic spine. Then widen your shoulder blades, and lengthen from your outer armpits to your inner elbows: this lengthens your cervical spine. Feel how the crown of your head rests lightly on the floor but your neck remains long and relaxed. Hold this position for 1 to 2 minutes; then lift your head, extend your arms, and either walk or spring your feet together. Return to Tadasana.

2.13b
*Prasarita Padottanasana,
Phase 2*

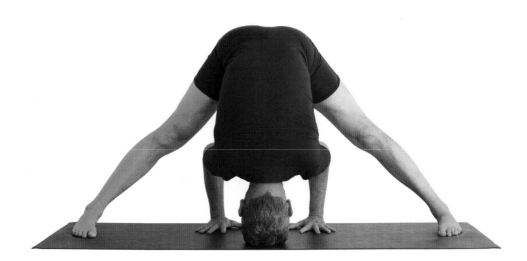

Practice Notes. If you are overly flexible, you may find that your head touches the floor easily, but you have no room to lengthen your spine. In this case, walk your feet closer together so that the crown of your head barely touches the floor. If your upper back feels rounded, take hold of your outer feet with your hands instead of placing your palms on the floor: this broadens your rib cage and lengthens your thoracic spine.

SALAMBA SIRSASANA AT THE WALL
HEADSTAND VARIATION

2.14
Salamba Sirsasana at the Wall

PROPS
- 1 wall
- set up as determined for Salamba Sirsasana earlier in this chapter

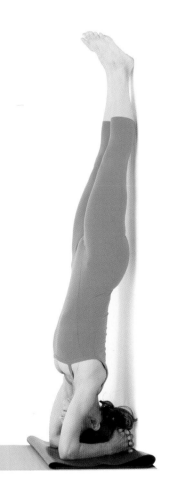

If you are unable to balance in the middle of the room, practice Salamba Sirsasana at the Wall (Figure 2.14). Place a folded blanket or folded mat at the base of a wall. (If using a folded blanket, place the blanket on a nonskid mat.) Then kneel in front of the blanket or mat, place your elbows in line with the center of your shoulder joints and interlock your fingers, so that your hands are almost touching the wall. Come into the pose with bent knees, as described for Salamba Sirsasana (Figure 2.1).

When using the wall for support, let your heels—but not your pelvis—rest on the wall. Draw your sacrum deeper into your body, lengthen your front thighs toward your knees, and slide your heels up the wall. When you rest your pelvis on the wall, the weight of your legs collapses onto your spine and your pose feels heavy. When you bring your pelvis away from the wall and activate your legs, your pose becomes lighter and balance comes more easily.

Practice Notes. If your feet rest on the wall in Salamba Sirsasana but your hands are several inches away from the wall, your chest may be overarched and your lumbar spine compressed. Place your hands close to the wall, so that your spine is more vertically aligned.

SALAMBA SIRSASANA NEAR THE WALL
HEADSTAND VARIATION

- 1 wall
- set up as determined for Salamba Sirsasana earlier in this chapter

2.15

Salamba Sirsasana near the Wall

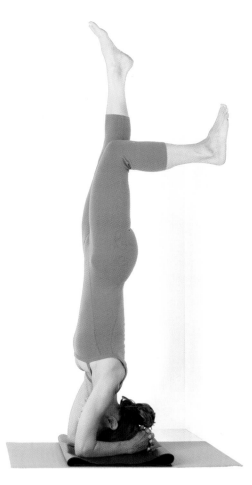

When you are able to balance away from the wall with a fair degree of confidence, but still feel apprehensive about practicing Salamba Sirsasana (Figure 2.1) in the middle of the room, try Salamba Sirsasana near the Wall (Figure 2.15) as an interim measure. Place your blanket or mat a few inches away from the wall, so that when you come into Salamba Sirsasana, your back is about 1½ feet away from the wall. In this way, you can gradually overcome your physical and psychological dependence on the wall.

Come into the pose either with bent knees or with straight legs, as described for Salamba Sirsasana.

In Salamba Sirsasana near the Wall, start with both feet resting on the wall, and bring your right leg away from the wall to a vertical position. Then press your lower sacrum deeper into your body, firm the core of your left buttock, and bring your left leg forward to meet your right leg. Maintain your balance for several breaths, then repeat this adjustment with your other leg. Keep your left leg lifting vertically, and bring your right foot back to the wall. Press your lower sacrum into your body, firm the core of your right buttock, and bring your right leg forward to meet your left leg. The strength of your legs will help you to balance.

Practice Notes. Practicing Salamba Sirsasana at the Wall (Figure 2.14) prevents you from overarching your back, because your hands are close to the wall; however, it also makes balancing more difficult. The wall sucks you into its orbit like a magnetic force. When you feel you have developed the necessary strength to balance, place your hands a few inches farther from the wall, and practice Salamba Sirsasana near the Wall to free yourself from the vortex and establish your independence.

SALAMBA SIRSASANA WITH BLOCKS AT THE WALL

HEADSTAND VARIATION

PROPS

- 1 nonskid mat
- 4 or 5 blocks
- 1 wall

If you have a kyphosis (rounded thoracic spine) or scoliosis (lateral curvature of the spine), or if the muscles of your upper back are very tight, practicing Salamba Sirsasana with Blocks at the Wall (Figure 2.16a) will give support to your upper back and allow your shoulder joints to open.

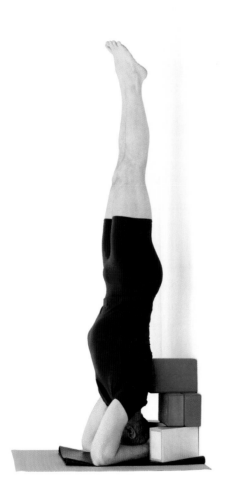

For this variation, fold a nonskid mat in half or in thirds to prevent your blocks from slipping. You will need four or five blocks, either wood or foam. First, arrange your mat at the base of a wall. Place two blocks on their sides on your mat in a V shape pointing toward the wall (Figure 2.16b). Make sure the blocks are identical in size and shape, with approximately a 60-degree angle between them. Stack another block flat on top of the first two blocks, with the long edge of the block touching the wall. (You may need to add a second block if you are tall or have a long spine.) Turn the final block on its side, with one end of the block touching the wall and the other end protruding into the room to support your upper back.

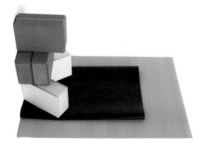

Position your elbows parallel to the front edge of your mat, interlock your fingers, and place your hands between the V-shaped blocks. Check that your hands are directly underneath the overhang of the topmost block. Widen your collarbones and place the crown of your head on the floor.

(Use a support under your head if appropriate.) Lift your knees and walk your feet, inch by inch, toward your mat until the overhanging block presses against your midthoracic spine. Keep your rib cage in firm contact with the block, and come into the pose by raising one leg at a time.

In Salamba Sirsasana with Blocks at the Wall, press your thoracic spine against the block, and lengthen your upper arms away from your elbows: this will widen your upper back and create space in your shoulder joints. Hold the pose for 1 to 3 minutes. When you are ready to come down, bend your knees, slide your feet down the wall, draw your thighs into your abdomen, and roll your pelvis away from the wall.

Practice Notes. If the block does not support your back at the appropriate place, your pose may feel awkward or unstable. As a general rule, the block should be in contact with your midthoracic spine. You may need to alter the height of your blocks to find the level that feels right for you. When you find an arrangement of blocks that works for you, make a note or drawing of it so that you don't forget.

▶
PRACTICE SUGGESTIONS

Timing Your Salamba Sirsasana. If you want to include Salamba Sirsasana (Figure 2.1) in your daily yoga routine, be consistent: practice the pose for the same amount of time each day. Use an electronic timer with a soft beep or a sports watch with a timing function to signal the end of the period. You can also place a watch or small clock in front of your blanket where you can see it easily, but this is more distracting.

Traditionally, in Iyengar-style yoga, Salamba Sirsasana is held by senior practitioners for 10 minutes. If you are a beginning student, however, you need to build your time in the pose gradually throughout a period of months or even years. Start with 1 or 2 minutes, and when you can hold Salamba Sirsasana comfortably for that length of time, add another 30 seconds or 1 minute. Spend another few weeks practicing for the increased amount of time and then reassess your pose. (See the section that follows, "Time for Reflection," for more suggestions.)

Do not turn Salamba Sirsasana into an endurance competition. If you reach a plateau of 5 or 6 minutes, and this feels adequate for you, there is no need to hold any longer. Listen to your body and work within the limits of your natural capacity. You can challenge yourself once a week or once a month by adding an additional 1 to 2 minutes. For maintaining a consistent home practice, however, find the length of time that allows you a sense of fullness and completion in the pose, without depleting your energy or creating tension or discomfort in your body.

If your home practice is interrupted for more than a few days, you may need to temporarily reduce the amount of time you hold Salamba Sirsasana once you resume your yoga routine. Do not immediately return to your previous level of practice, especially if you are recovering from illness, injury, or the effects of travel. Reduce your holding time by about one-third until you regain your strength and stamina.

Time for Reflection. Take a few moments after practicing Salamba Sirsasana (Figure 2.1) to observe the physiological effects of the pose, particularly, the state of your mind. As your practice matures, you will find that Salamba Sirsasana leaves you feeling calm yet alert, inwardly poised yet outwardly looking. This mental state is unique to Salamba Sirsasana and one of its chief benefits.

Pay attention to the anatomical effects of the pose as well. Do not let a minor irritation grow into a major problem. If you feel stiffness or tension in your neck or shoulders, include one or two poses that bring you relief, such as Adho Mukha Svanasana (Figure 3.4a) or Bharadvajasana (Figure 6.16).

If you feel discomfort whenever you practice Salamba Sirsasana, seek the advice of an experienced yoga teacher. You may need to change the position of your head, the cup of your hands, or the height of your props. Consult your teacher as soon as you become aware of the problem, not six months down the road.

If you experience occasional discomfort, can you determine an immediate or probable cause? What have you been doing besides yoga? Picking up your child, gardening overzealously, or sleeping on your shoulder? What other asana did you practice before Salamba Sirsasana, and how did they affect your body? The way you sequence your practice can make Salamba Sirsasana feel easier or more difficult. For suggestions on how to sequence Salamba Sirsasana most effectively, read the following section.

▶
SEQUENCING YOUR PRACTICE

In sequencing Salamba Sirsasana (Figure 2.1) in your practice, you need to consider both the anatomical and the physiological aspects of the pose. What poses are useful to practice before Salamba Sirsasana to open your shoulders, strengthen your lower abdomen, and prepare your body physically? What poses are effective counterposes to practice after Salamba Sirsasana to release any tension or discomfort?

At the physiological level, how does Salamba Sirsasana affect you energetically? Does it feel more difficult and dynamic in the morning, but more calming and restorative in the afternoon? How you sequence Salamba Sirsasana depends on a variety of factors: the time of day, your body type, and the other poses you intend to practice.

First, consider what poses to practice immediately before and immediately after Salamba Sirsasana. Immediately before Salamba Sirsasana, practice Adho Mukha Svanasana (Figure 3.4a) or Uttanasana (Figure 3.7) for at least 1 minute to bring your heart lower than your head and prepare you physiologically for the pose. Immediately after Salamba Sirsasana, rest in Adho Mukha Virasana (Child's Pose, Figure 3.11b) for 30 seconds before proceeding.

Then consider how Salamba Sirsasana fits into the theme of your practice. Here are some general guidelines for sequencing Salamba Sirsasana in relation to different types of poses: standing poses, backbends, sitting twists, sitting forward bends, and, in particular, Salamba Sarvangasana (Figure 1.1).

Standing Poses. Practice Salamba Sirsasana after standing poses. Standing poses help to warm your body and lubricate your joints. The pose will feel easier after standing poses, especially if you practice in the morning.

Backbends. Practice Salamba Sirsasana either before or after backbends, depending on your body type. On the one hand, if you have tightness in your shoulders and upper back, Salamba Sirsasana will feel easier and more balanced when practiced after backbends. On the other hand, if you are very flexible, you may find that your Salamba Sirsasana feels weak and unstable after a series of backbends. In this case, it is safer and more effective for you to practice Salamba Sirsasana before backbends.

Sitting Twists. Sitting twists are excellent transition poses because they balance, or neutralize, your spine. You can practice them beneficially either before or after Salamba Sirsasana. Sitting twists act as preparatory poses when practiced before Salamba Sirsasana because they develop flexibility in your shoulders and strengthen your lower abdomen. Sitting twists also function as counterposes when practiced after Salamba Sirsasana because they release stiffness and discomfort in your neck, shoulders, and upper back.

Sitting Forward Bends. Practice Salamba Sirsasana before sitting forward bends. These poses calm your nervous system and pacify your mind. Salamba Sirsasana can feel heavy and lack vital energy when practiced after sitting forward bends.

Salamba Sarvangasana. You can practice Salamba Sarvangasana without practicing Salamba Sirsasana. If you practice Salamba Sirsasana, however, be sure to include some variation of Salamba Sarvangasana, either directly after Salamba Sirsasana or later in your sequence. Whereas Salamba Sirsasana tends to compress your neck, Salamba Sarvangasana is an ideal counterpose because it releases and lengthens your cervical spine.

You will feel much more stable and be less vulnerable to injury in both of these poses if you practice them daily (or nearly every day) for the same length of time each day. Once you add Salamba Sirsasana and Salamba Sarvangasana to your home yoga practice, include them on a regular basis.

PART 2:

Themes and
Variations

3 THE THREE DIAPHRAGMS

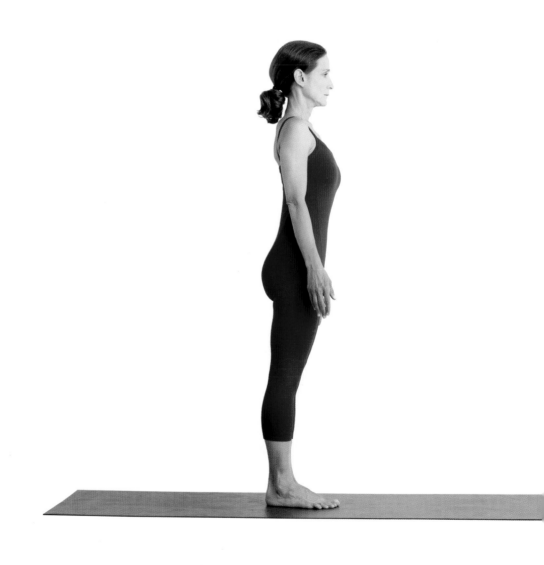

IN THIS CHAPTER, we explore the nature and function of the three dia-phragms: the pelvic diaphragm, the respiratory diaphragm, and the thoracic inlet; in the yoga tradition, the thoracic inlet is known as the thoracic diaphragm. The word *diaphragm* derives from the Greek *dia,* meaning "through," "across," or "apart," and *phragma,* meaning "fence." A diaphragm is, therefore, primarily something that sep-arates and contains or creates a border.

The three diaphragms are cross-sections that divide the body into vertical seg-ments. The pelvic diaphragm marks the juncture between the legs and pelvis; the res-piratory diaphragm divides the abdominal and thoracic cavities; and the thoracic diaphragm separates the thoracic cavity from the shoulder girdle, arms, and cervical region (Figure 3.1).

In Tadasana (Figure 3.3), you can visualize a flat, circular plane passing through the circumference of each diaphragm to develop your awareness of the horizontal planes of the body. When all three diaphragms are parallel to the floor and stacked in con-centric planes, then your pelvis, rib cage, and shoulder girdle are properly aligned (Figure 3.2).

In general, broadening in the horizontal plane neutralizes tension and creates space in the body. Widening the pelvic diaphragm creates space in the hip joints. Broaden-

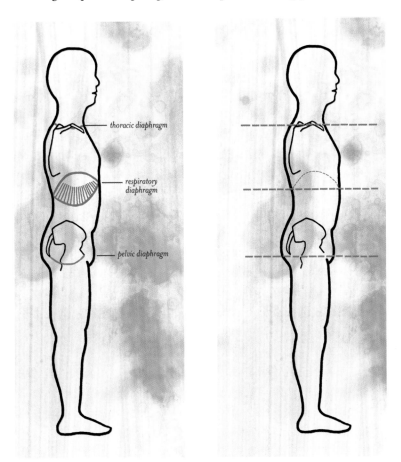

thoracic diaphragm

respiratory diaphragm

pelvic diaphragm

3.1
The Three Diaphragms

3.2
The Planes of the Diaphragms

ing the respiratory diaphragm creates space between the lungs and the abdominal organs, in particular, the liver and stomach. Widening the thoracic diaphragm creates space between the rib cage and shoulder girdle, and allows the shoulder joints to open.

In contrast, creating space *between* the diaphragms vertically helps to lengthen the spine. For example, in Adho Mukha Svanasana (Figure 3.4a), lifting the pelvic diaphragm away from the respiratory diaphragm releases the lumbar spine; lifting the respiratory diaphragm away from the thoracic diaphragm lengthens the thoracic spine; and lifting the sides of the thoracic diaphragm away from the arms releases the cervical spine.

Ideally, your pelvic, respiratory, and thoracic diaphragms will not only be properly aligned with one another, but also will be comparable in tone and quality. In Virabhadrasana II (Figure 4.7), for example, your three diaphragms may all be parallel to the floor, and yet your pelvic diaphragm may be broad and elastic, your respiratory diaphragm loose and slack, and your thoracic diaphragm narrow and constricted. In this case, to balance the pose energetically, keep your pelvic diaphragm broad, firm your respiratory diaphragm, and soften and widen your thoracic diaphragm, so that the strength and tone of all three diaphragms feels more equal.

The broadening of the pelvic, respiratory, and thoracic diaphragms is experienced less as a muscular action, and more as a release of connective tissue in the horizontal plane. As you work with the practice sequence in this chapter, learn to distinguish between a muscular sensation, such as lifting the perineum, and the elastic stretch of connective tissue that comes with broadening the pelvic diaphragm.

A diaphragm is not a solid partition, but a taut, flexible membrane that transmits vibrations like the skin of a drum. Because of its elastic nature, each of the diaphragms plays a significant role in breathing. The pelvic diaphragm governs the movement of breath in the lower abdomen. The respiratory diaphragm controls the flow of breath in the lower and middle lungs, while the lifting action of the thoracic diaphragm draws the breath gently into the upper lungs.

Pelvic Diaphragm. The base of the pelvis is composed of horizontal layers of muscles and connective tissue that support the abdominal organs like slings. The outermost layer is the perineum, the diamond-shaped area defined by the tailbone, the sitting bones, and the pubic symphysis (the cartilage joining the two sides of the pubic bone).

The pelvic diaphragm is directly above the perineum, and consists of the muscles of the pelvic floor and their connective tissue. Anatomically, the pelvic diaphragm is funnel shaped, but I find it helpful to imagine a flat circular plane that intersects with the circumference of the pelvic diaphragm and lies parallel to the floor. The center of the pelvic diaphragm is directly above the center of the perineum, and the circumference of the pelvic diaphragm is in line with the center of the hip joints.

The proper alignment of your pelvis depends upon establishing a balance between broadening your pelvic diaphragm and lifting your perineum. How you achieve this balance depends on your body type. If your hip joints are tight, your pelvic diaphragm will be narrow and restricted. As you practice the sequence in this chapter, focus on broadening the circumference of your pelvic diaphragm to create space in your hip joints. If your hip joints are overly flexible and you need to build strength and stability, focus on lifting the center of your perineum into your body.

Respiratory Diaphragm. Composed of skeletal muscle and dense connective tissue, the respiratory diaphragm separates the abdominal and thoracic cavities. At the back of the body, the diaphragm attaches to the first three lumbar vertebrae (L1–L3); at the sides, to the cartilage and bone of the lower six ribs; and at the front of the body, to the xiphoid process. The diaphragm is the prime mover of the breath: the contraction of the diaphragm stimulates the expansion of the lungs in respiration.

Anatomically, the diaphragm is dome shaped, like a jellyfish. As with the pelvic diaphragm, however, I find it helpful to visualize a horizontal plane that intersects the circumference of the respiratory diaphragm and passes through the thoraco-lumbar joint at the back of the body, and the tip of the xiphoid process at the front of the body. When your pelvis and rib cage are properly aligned in Tadasana, the plane of your respiratory diaphragm will be parallel to the floor, and the center of your respiratory diaphragm will be directly over the center of your perineum.

Thoracic Diaphragm. The thoracic diaphragm, which separates the thoracic cavity from the cervical region, is much smaller than the respiratory diaphragm. The thoracic diaphragm is sometimes called the *operculum*, which means "lid" in Latin. It is composed of the soft tissues that attach onto the first ribs, collarbones, and the body of the first thoracic vertebra (T1), including the suspensory ligaments that attach directly onto the pleural dome (the covering of the upper lungs). The thoracic diaphragm is known anatomically as the thoracic inlet because the blood and lymphatic vessels that pass through this opening are profoundly affected by the movement and changing shape of this diaphragm during respiration.

As with the other two diaphragms, when standing in Tadasana, you can visualize the thoracic diaphragm as a flat, circular plane parallel to the floor. The front edge of the thoracic diaphragm lies behind your collarbones, and the back edge is parallel to the top edges of your shoulder blades. The sides of your thoracic diaphragm are parallel to the sides of your neck. When your arms are raised overhead, as in Virabhadrasana I (Figure 3.10) or Adho Mukha Svanasana, the plane of the thoracic diaphragm passes through the center of your shoulder joints. Just as the broadening of your pelvic diaphragm creates space in your hip joints, the broadening of your thoracic diaphragm creates space in your shoulder joints.

In the following sequence of poses, you learn how to balance each of the three diaphragms—both individually and in relation to one another. By adjusting the diaphragms, you improve your alignment, help to create space in your joints, and lengthen your spine. You observe whether a diaphragm is too slack or too tight, and use your awareness to modify the tone and quality of each diaphragm. Finally, you explore the effect of each of the diaphragms on your breath with some simple breathing practices.

TADASANA
MOUNTAIN POSE

PROP

• 1 nonskid mat

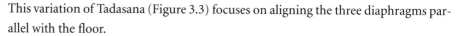

This variation of Tadasana (Figure 3.3) focuses on aligning the three diaphragms parallel with the floor.

Stand on your mat in Tadasana with your feet together, and your arms extended by your sides. Adjust your pelvis so that your pelvic diaphragm is parallel to the floor, and the center of your perineum is directly below the center of your respiratory diaphragm. If your hips are tight, widen the circumference of your pelvic diaphragm in all directions, so that you feel more space in your hip joints. If your hips are flexible, lift the front edge of your pelvic diaphragm from behind your pubic bone, and draw the center of your perineum into your body to strengthen and stabilize your pelvis.

Then bring your respiratory diaphragm parallel to the floor, directly over your pelvic diaphragm. Broaden the back edge of your respiratory diaphragm, and lift the sides of your rib cage vertically. At the same time, lift your xiphoid process away from the front edge of your respiratory diaphragm and broaden your midsternum.

3.3
Tadasana

Now widen your collarbones and relax your shoulder blades. Lift the front edge of your thoracic diaphragm toward the base of your throat, but keep the back edge of your thoracic diaphragm broad. Lengthen the back of your arms away from the sides of your thoracic diaphragm. Soften the skin of your face, and draw your eyes deeper into their sockets. Return to this position between each of the standing poses.

RELATED POSE. Virabhadrasana II

ADHO MUKHA SVANASANA
DOWNWARD-FACING DOG POSE

PROP
- 1 nonskid mat

This variation of Adho Mukha Svanasana (Figure 3.4a) focuses on aligning the three diaphragms to lengthen the spine, and to create space in the hip and shoulder joints.

Begin on your mat in Adho Mukha Virasana with Arms Extended (Child's Pose Variation, Figure 3.4b), with your pelvis resting on your heels and your arms extended forward. Place your hands on the mat with the mounds of your thumbs in line with the center of your shoulder joints; broaden your palms. Then come to a kneeling position so that your knees and your feet are in line with the center of your hip joints. With an inhalation, curl your toes under. With an exhalation, lift your pelvis and straighten your legs.

In Adho Mukha Svanasana, widen the back edge of your pelvic diaphragm, and lift it away from the back edge of your respiratory diaphragm to lengthen your lumbar spine. At the same time, lift the front edge of your pelvic diaphragm toward your inner thighs to bring the plane of your pelvic diaphragm in line with the back of your legs. Then lengthen your hamstrings, widen the back edge of your pelvic diaphragm, and draw the center of your perineum into your body to strengthen your pelvic floor.

3.4a
Adho Mukha Svanasana

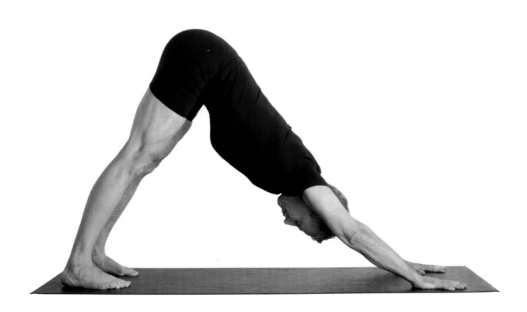

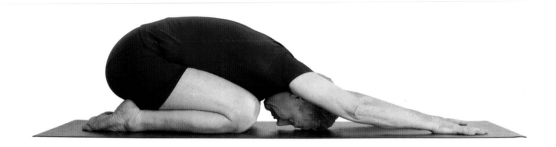

3.4b
Adho Mukha Virasana
with Arms Extended

Next, widen the back edge of your respiratory diaphragm, and lift it away from the back edge of your thoracic diaphragm to release your thoracic spine. Lengthen the back of your rib cage toward your arms, and turn your xiphoid process toward your navel to bring your respiratory diaphragm parallel to your pelvic diaphragm. Finally, lift the sides of your pelvis away from the sides of your respiratory diaphragm to lengthen the sides of your waist.

Now widen the back edge of your thoracic diaphragm, and move it toward your shoulders to release your cervical spine. Turn the front edge of your thoracic diaphragm away from the base of your throat, and lengthen the front of your rib cage toward your xiphoid process to bring your thoracic diaphragm parallel to your respiratory diaphragm. Then lift the sides of your thoracic diaphragm away from your arms to create space in your shoulder joints and bring more weight onto your legs.

Hold this position for 1 to 2 minutes, observing the alignment of your three diaphragms. Lift your pelvic diaphragm away from your respiratory diaphragm; lift your respiratory diaphragm away from your thoracic diaphragm; and lift your thoracic diaphragm away from your arms. Allow your spine to lengthen. Observe the tone and quality of each of your three diaphragms. If one diaphragm is tighter than the others, soften the circumference of that diaphragm and let it expand. If one diaphragm is much looser than the others, strengthen the circumference of that diaphragm. When you are ready to come out of the pose, bend your knees and return to Adho Mukha Virasana with Arms Extended.

UTTHITA PARSVAKONASANA
EXTENDED SIDE-ANGLE POSE

PROP
• 1 nonskid mat

OPTIONAL PROP
• 1 block

In Utthita Parsvakonasana (Figure 3.5), the pelvic diaphragm stays parallel to the floor, but the respiratory diaphragm moves perpendicular to the floor to maximize the stretch at the side of the waist.

Stand on your mat in Tadasana (Figure 3.3), place your hands on your hips, and step your feet about 4 to 4½ feet apart. Turn your left foot in 30 degrees and your right foot out 90 degrees. Bring your pelvic diaphragm parallel to the floor, so that the center of your perineum is directly below the center of your respiratory diaphragm and your hipbones are level. With an inhalation, widen your thoracic diaphragm and raise your arms out to the sides to shoulder level. With an exhalation, keep your pelvic diaphragm broad as you bend your right knee to a right angle, and place your right hand on the floor by your outer right ankle. (If your right hand does not reach the floor, use a block under your hand.) Then swing your left arm overhead, in line with your outer left rib cage, and let your palm face down.

In Utthita Parsvakonasana, bring the center of your perineum in line with the center of your respiratory diaphragm to align your pelvis and rib cage. Then widen your pelvic diaphragm to create more space in your hip joints. Lift the left side of your respiratory diaphragm away from the left side of your pelvic diaphragm to lengthen the left side of your lumbar spine and waist.

Then lift the left side of your thoracic diaphragm away from the left side of your respiratory diaphragm; this lengthens the left side of your rib cage and creates space in your left shoulder joint. Lift the front edge of your thoracic diaphragm toward the base of your throat, draw your seventh cervical vertebra (C7) deeper into your body, and let your head drop gently back. Remain in this position for another 30 seconds, and then repeat to the other side.

RELATED POSE. Virabhadrasana II

3.5
Utthita Parsvakonasana

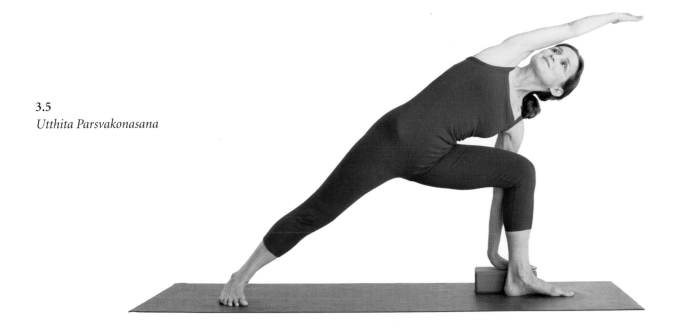

PADANGUSTHASANA
TOE-HOLDING POSE

PROP
- 1 nonskid mat

OPTIONAL PROP
- 1 block

This variation of Padangusthasana (Figure 3.6) focuses on the accordionlike movement of the three diaphragms away from one another, which creates maximum length in the spine.

Stand on your mat in Tadasana (Figure 3.3) with your feet parallel and a few inches apart. Place your hands on your hips with your thumbs pressing the top edge of your sacrum, and press your elbows toward each other, so that your upper arms are parallel. With an inhalation, press your thumbs down on your sacrum as you lift the back edge of your respiratory diaphragm away from the top edge of your sacrum. At the same time, lift the front edge of your thoracic diaphragm toward the base of your throat, and let your head drop back.

With an exhalation, draw your groins into your body and lift your pelvis over your thighbones as you come into the forward bend. When your torso is parallel to the floor, extend your arms and wrap your second and third fingers around your big toes. (If you cannot reach your big toes without rounding your back, place a block on end in front of your feet, and rest your hands on the block.)

3.6
Padangusthasana

3.7
Uttanasana

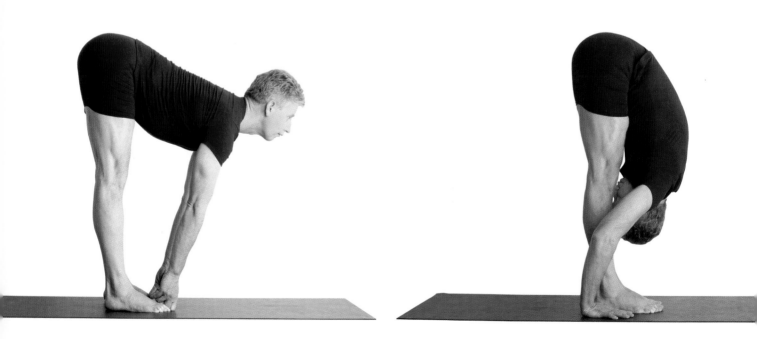

In Padangusthasana, lift your pelvic diaphragm vertically away from the back of your thighs and lengthen your hamstrings. Let the circumference of your pelvic diaphragm expand in all directions, especially if you are tight in your hip joints. If you are overly flexible in your hip joints, draw the center of your perineum into your body to strengthen and stabilize your pelvis.

Press the top edge of your sacrum toward your legs, and lift the back edge of your respiratory diaphragm toward your shoulders to release your lumbar spine. Then lift your xiphoid process and turn the front edge of your thoracic diaphragm toward your head to lengthen your thoracic spine. Finally, lift the base of your skull away from your C7, and soften the skin of your face. Maintain this position for several breaths, and then move into Uttanasana (Figure 3.7) from Padangusthasana, as in the following section.

RELATED POSE. Prasarita Padottanasana (Phase 1)

UTTANASANA
STANDING FORWARD BEND

PROP
• 1 nonskid mat

OPTIONAL PROP
• 1 block

In Uttanasana (Figure 3.7), the pelvic diaphragm lifts vertically and the respiratory diaphragm comes parallel to the floor.

Start on your mat in Padangusthasana, as shown in Figure 3.6. With an inhalation, draw the center of your perineum into your body, and lengthen your spine through the crown of your head. With an exhalation, bend your elbows and bring your midsternum toward your thighs to come into Uttanasana. Place your hands by the sides of your feet with your upper arms parallel to each other; release your head so that it hangs freely. (If your hands do not reach the floor, place a block in front of your feet, and rest your hands on the block.)

In Uttanasana, lift your pelvic diaphragm away from the back of your thighs and lengthen your hamstrings. Let the circumference of your pelvic diaphragm expand in all directions, especially if you have tight hip joints. If you have flexible hip joints, draw the center of your perineum deeper into your body.

Then soften and broaden the back edge of your respiratory diaphragm, and move it down toward your shoulders. At the same time, gently turn your xiphoid process toward your navel, so that your respiratory diaphragm comes parallel to the floor. Now soften and broaden the back edge of your thoracic diaphragm. Turn the front edge of your thoracic diaphragm toward your rib cage, but move the back edge of your thoracic diaphragm toward your shoulders. Lift the sides of your thoracic diaphragm away from your neck, and release the weight of your head.

Remain in this position for another 30 seconds. Balance the tone and quality of all three diaphragms. To come out of the pose, raise your head, lift from the strength of your upper spine, and return to Tadasana (Figure 3.3).

RELATED POSE. Prasarita Padottanasana (Phase 2)

ARDHA CHANDRASANA
HALF-MOON POSE

PROP	OPTIONAL PROP
• 1 nonskid mat	• 1 block

3.8
Ardha Chandrasana

In Ardha Chandrasana (Figure 3.8), the pelvic diaphragm is aligned vertically with the hamstrings of the standing leg.

Stand on your mat in Tadasana (Figure 3.3), and bring your feet approximately 3 to 3½ feet apart. Turn your left foot in 30 degrees and your right foot out 90 degrees. With an inhalation, widen your thoracic diaphragm as you raise your arms to shoulder level. With an exhalation, bend your right knee, lift your left heel off the floor, and place the fingertips of your right hand on the floor directly beneath your right shoulder. (If your hamstrings are tight or your balance is unsteady, use a block to support your hand.) With an inhalation, bring the center of your perineum in line with the center of your respiratory diaphragm and open your chest. With an exhalation, lift your pelvic diaphragm away from your hamstrings as you straighten your right leg.

In Ardha Chandrasana, check that the center of your perineum is in line with the center of your respiratory diaphragm. Lift your pelvic diaphragm away from the hamstrings of your standing leg, until you feel the stretch of the connective tissue. If your pelvic diaphragm is tight, allow the circumference to broaden in all directions. If your pelvic diaphragm is weak, lift the center of your perineum away from the tip of your tailbone to strengthen your pelvic floor. (Make this adjustment slowly and gradually, so that you do not throw yourself off balance!)

Maintain this position for 30 seconds. Lift the left side of your respiratory diaphragm away from the left side of your pelvic diaphragm; simultaneously, lift the right side of your rib cage away from the floor. Then widen the back edge of your thoracic diaphragm, and lift the front edge of your thoracic diaphragm toward the base of your throat. Draw your C7 into your body to release your neck.

To come out of the pose, keep the center of your perineum in line with the center of your respiratory diaphragm as you bend your right knee and lower your left leg. Then straighten your right leg and lift your torso return to a standing position. Repeat to the other side.

RELATED POSE. Utthita Trikonasana

PARIVRTTA ARDHA CHANDRASANA AT THE WALL
REVOLVED HALF-MOON POSE

PROPS
- 1 nonskid mat
- 1 wall

OPTIONAL PROP
- 1 block

In Parivrtta Ardha Chandrasana at the Wall (Figure 3.9), the pelvic diaphragm remains stable while the respiratory diaphragm revolves up to 90 degrees.

Stand on your mat in Tadasana (Figure 3.3) with your left side facing a wall. Separate your feet 3 to 3½ feet apart, with the outer edge of your left foot touching the base of the wall. Turn your left foot in 60 degrees so that your outer heel is in contact with the wall, and turn your right foot out 90 degrees, in line with your left heel. Place your hands onto your hips with your thumbs pressing the top edge of your sacrum. Then

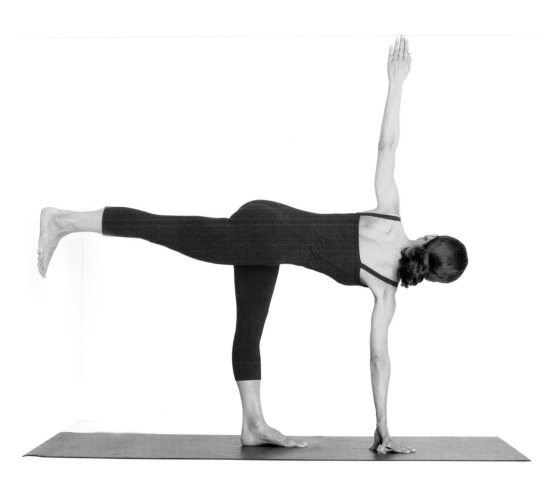

3.9

Parivrtta Ardha Chandrasana at the Wall

draw your right groin back into your body, and from the center of your perineum, turn your pelvis to face your right leg.

With an inhalation, raise your left arm overhead. Then turn and lift from the left side of your respiratory diaphragm, and lengthen the left side of your rib cage. With an exhalation, bend your right knee, shift your weight onto your right foot, and place the fingertips of your left hand on the floor directly below your left shoulder. (If your hamstrings are tight or your balance is unsteady, use a block to support your hand.) With another inhalation, straighten your right leg and place your left foot on the wall with your toes pointing down, so that your left leg and spine are parallel to the floor. With an exhalation, bring the center of your perineum in line with the center of your respiratory diaphragm and lengthen your spine.

In Parivrtta Ardha Chandrasana at the Wall, lift your pelvic diaphragm away from the hamstrings of your standing leg, and lengthen your raised leg from the center of your perineum. To deepen the twist, turn the left side of your respiratory diaphragm toward the right side of your pelvic diaphragm. At the same time, widen the back edge of your thoracic diaphragm by lengthening your arms, and lift the front edge of your thoracic diaphragm toward the base of your throat. Check that the crown of your head is in line with your tailbone.

Maintain this position for 30 seconds, focusing on the alignment of your three diaphragms. To lengthen your lumbar spine, lift the right side of your respiratory diaphragm away from the right side of your pelvic diaphragm. To release your thoracic spine, lift the right side of your thoracic diaphragm away from the right side of your respiratory diaphragm. Then draw your C7 into your body to release your cervical spine. When you are ready to come out of the pose, bend your right knee and bring your left foot back to the floor at the base of the wall. Repeat to the other side.

RELATED POSE. Parivrtta Trikonasana

VIRABHADRASANA I
WARRIOR POSE I

PROP
• 1 nonskid mat

3.10
Virabhadrasana I

In Virabhadrasana I (Figure 3.10), your pelvic diaphragm stays parallel to the floor, the back edge of your respiratory diaphragm lifts up, and the front edge of your thoracic diaphragm turns toward the base of your throat.

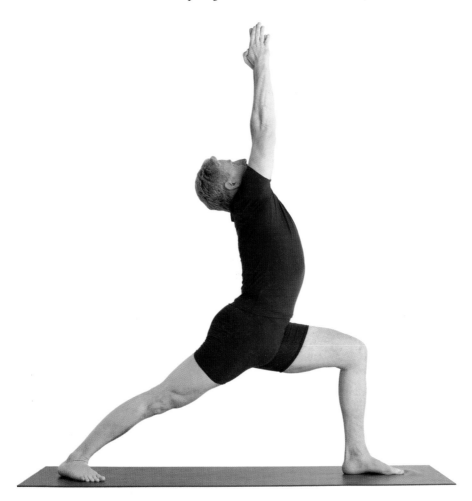

Stand on your mat in Tadasana (Figure 3.3) and separate your legs 4 to 4½ feet apart, with your feet parallel. Turn your left foot in 30 degrees and your right foot out 90 degrees. Draw your right groin back into your body, and from the center of your perineum, turn your pelvis to face your right leg. Then place your hands on your hips, and bring your elbows together so that your upper arms are parallel.

With your thumbs pressing down on your sacrum, lift the back edge of your respiratory diaphragm away from the top edge of your sacrum. At the same time, turn the front edge of your thoracic diaphragm toward the base of your throat, and lift from the sides of your chest. If it feels comfortable on your neck, you can let your head drop back and lift your C7 into your body. Then, with an inhalation, raise your arms overhead and lift from the sides of your thoracic diaphragm. With an exhalation, keep your pelvic diaphragm parallel to the floor as you bend your right knee over your right heel.

In Virabhadrasana I, stretch your pelvic diaphragm from the center of your left hip joint toward your right knee, broadening the circumference in all directions. If your pelvis tilts forward and your lower back arches, you may be compressing your lumbar spine. In this case, lift the front edge of your pelvic diaphragm from behind your pubic bone and lengthen your lumbar spine. Then lift your xiphoid process away from the front edge of your respiratory diaphragm to release your thoracic spine. Finally, turn the front edge of your thoracic diaphragm toward the base of your throat to relax your cervical spine.

Maintain this position for 30 seconds, observing the alignment and balance of your three diaphragms. Then come out of the pose, and repeat to the other side.

ADHO MUKHA VRKSASANA AT THE WALL
HANDSTAND

PROPS
• 1 nonskid mat   • 1 wall

In this variation of Adho Mukha Vrksasana at the Wall (Figure 3.11a), first, adjust your pelvic diaphragm; then adjust your respiratory diaphragm; and finally, adjust your thoracic diaphragm.

Spread your nonskid mat lengthwise at the base of a wall. Start in Adho Mukha Svanasana (Figure 3.4a) with your hands about 6 inches from the wall. Lift the back

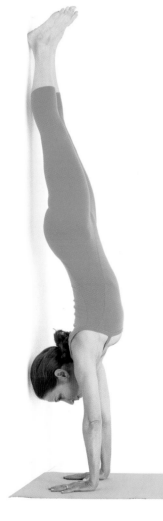

3.11a
Adho Mukha Vrksasana at the Wall

edge of your pelvic diaphragm away from the back edge of your respiratory diaphragm, and lift the sides of your thoracic diaphragm away from your arms. Then bring your shoulders directly over your hands, keeping your thoracic diaphragm broad. Bend one leg and step your foot in closer to your chest. Keep your other leg straight and strong as you swing it toward the wall. Let the momentum of your straight leg draw your bent leg away from the floor.

In Adho Mukha Vrksasana at the Wall, extend your heels up the wall, but move the center of your perineum away from your tailbone, so that your pelvis comes away from the wall. Then broaden your pelvic diaphragm, and lift the center of your perineum toward your legs. Relax the floating ribs at the front of your body, and move the back edge of your respiratory diaphragm toward your arms. At the same time, turn your xiphoid process toward your navel, and lift from the sides of your chest.

Now move the back edge of your thoracic diaphragm toward your shoulders, but lift the sides of your thoracic diaphragm away from your arms to create space in your shoulder joints. Finally, turn the front edge of your thoracic diaphragm toward the base of your throat as you lengthen your neck and lift your head. Remain in this position for 30 seconds. Keep the back edge of your respiratory diaphragm broad as you bring your legs down. Rest in Adho Mukha Virasana (Child's Pose, Figure 3.11b) or Uttanasana (Figure 3.7) until your breath returns to normal.

RELATED POSE. Pincha Mayurasana

3.11b
Adho Mukha Virasana

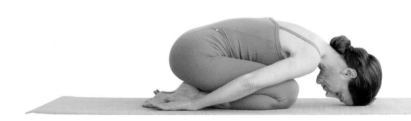

USTRASANA
CAMEL POSE

PROPS
- 1 nonskid mat
- 1 blanket

OPTIONAL PROPS
- 1 block
- 1 bolster

In Ustrasana (Figure 3.12), your pelvic diaphragm stays parallel to the floor, and your respiratory diaphragm and thoracic diaphragm turn toward your head.

Place a folded blanket on your nonskid mat. Then kneel on your blanket with your hip joints directly over your knees. (Use a block lengthwise between your feet to keep them apart, if you find it helpful.) Place your hands on your hips, with your thumbs pressing down on the top edge of your sacrum. Lift the back edge of your respiratory diaphragm away from the top edge of your sacrum to avoid compression of your lumbar spine. At the same time, lift the sides of your rib cage, and narrow your back floating ribs. Then let your head drop back, and bring your hands onto your feet with your arms extended. (If you cannot reach your heels or if you experience discomfort in your lower back, place a bolster across your lower legs to support your hands. If you have neck problems, keep your chin tucked into your chest.)

In Ustrasana, check that your pelvic diaphragm is parallel to the floor. If you tend to tilt your pelvis forward, the back edge of your pelvic diaphragm may be higher than the front edge. In this case, lift the front edge of your pelvic diaphragm away from your pubic bone to align your pelvic diaphragm. If you tuck your tailbone under, the front edge of your pelvic diaphragm will be higher than the back edge. In this event, move the front edge of your pelvic diaphragm toward your pubic bone to bring your pelvic diaphragm parallel to the floor.

When your pelvic diaphragm is stable, lift the back edge of your respiratory diaphragm away from the top edge of your sacrum, and turn your xiphoid process toward your head. Then widen and draw the back edge of your thoracic diaphragm away from your shoulders; turn the front edge toward the base of your throat. Lift your C7 deeper into your body to release your head and neck.

Remain in Ustrasana for 30 seconds. Keep your pelvic diaphragm parallel to the floor, but lift and turn your respiratory diaphragm and thoracic diaphragm toward your head. Balance the tone and quality of all three diaphragms to move deeper into the pose.

3.12
Ustrasana

To come out of Ustrasana, turn your xiphoid process toward your navel, and drop your chin toward your chest. Then sit back on your heels, with your hands on your thighs, and let your breathing return to normal. Repeat this pose two or three times.

RELATED POSES. Urdhva Mukha Svanasana, other backbends

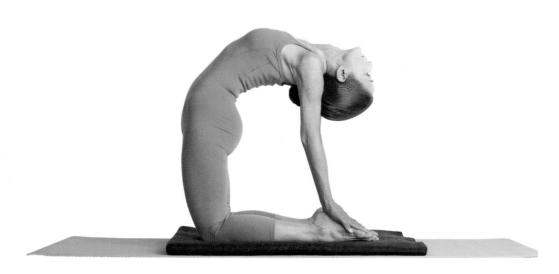

URDHVA DHANURASANA
UPWARD-FACING BOW POSE

PROP
- 1 nonskid mat
- 2 blocks
- 1 wedge

OPTIONAL PROP
- 1 chair

The following instructions apply to any variation of Urdhva Dhanurasana (Figure 3.13), either with your hands supported by a wedge or blocks, or with your feet elevated on blocks or a chair. If your shoulders are tight and you have difficulty contacting your thoracic diaphragm, you may find it helpful to practice this pose with your feet elevated.

Lie on your back with your knees bent and your feet in line with your sitting bones, about 2 or 3 inches forward of the sitting bones. Bend your elbows, and place your palms on the floor by the sides of your head, shoulder-width apart. Lengthen from the bottom tips of your shoulder blades to your elbows, so that your upper arms are parallel. With an inhalation, relax your shoulder girdle. With an exhalation, lift from the back edge of your respiratory diaphragm to come into the pose.

In Urdhva Dhanurasana, lift the back edge of your respiratory diaphragm away from the top edge of your sacrum to lengthen your lumbar spine. As you lift the back edge of your respiratory diaphragm, narrow your back floating ribs, and turn your xiphoid process toward your head. At the same time, lengthen your front thighs toward your knees, and draw the center of your perineum into your body.

3.13
Urdhva Dhanurasana

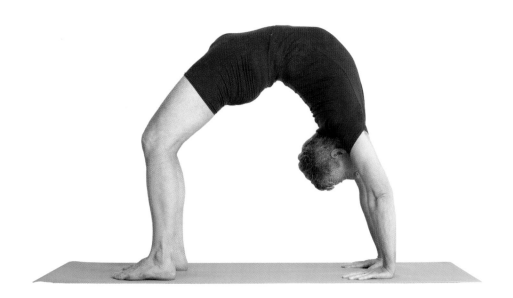

Now bring your thoracic diaphragm parallel to the floor. Start by relaxing your shoulder blades and widening your thoracic diaphragm. Then draw the back edge of your thoracic diaphragm away from your shoulders, and turn the front edge of your thoracic diaphragm toward the base of your throat. At the same time, lift the sides of your thoracic diaphragm away from your inner elbows.

Remain in Urdhva Dhanurasana for 30 seconds. Lift the back edge of your respiratory diaphragm, draw the center of your perineum into your body, and turn the front edge of your thoracic diaphragm toward your head. When you come down, rest with your back on the floor until your breathing returns to normal. Repeat the pose three to six times. It gets easier each time!

RELATED POSE. Viparita Dandasana

MARICHYASANA III
POSE OF SAGE MARICHI III

PROPS
- 1 nonskid mat
- 1 blanket

In Marichyasana III (Figure 3.14), turn from the back of your body, and keep the front of your body soft and broad, so that your breathing is not restricted.

Begin by folding a standard folded blanket in thirds, so that it measures about 6 inches wide and 3 or 4 inches high. Place the blanket lengthwise on your mat. Then sit with your sitting bones on the narrow edge of the blanket with your legs extended. Bend your right knee and place your right foot on the floor with your heel close to

3.14
Marichyasana III

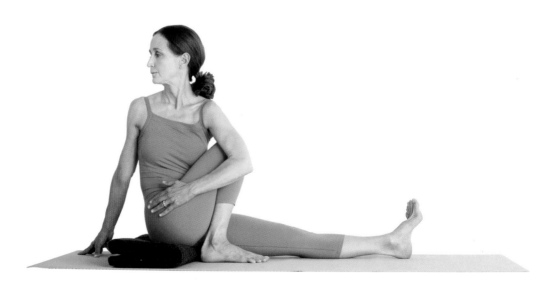

your right sitting bone. Take hold of your right knee with your left hand, and lean back onto your right arm. Lengthen from your left groin to your right shoulder as you turn your lower abdomen to the right, and bring your left arm to the outside of your right leg. Then lengthen your spine away from your sitting bones.

In Marichyasana III, lift the front edge of your pelvic diaphragm away from your pubic bone, and drop the back edge of your pelvic diaphragm toward the floor. To deepen the twist in your lower abdomen, turn from the back edge of your pelvic diaphragm by extending through your left leg.

Then bring your awareness to your respiratory diaphragm. Keep the front edge of your respiratory diaphragm soft and broad, and turn from the back edge. To deepen the twist in your upper abdomen, turn the left side of your respiratory diaphragm toward the right side of your pelvic diaphragm, and lift the right side of your respiratory diaphragm away from the left side of your pelvic diaphragm. Bring your xiphoid process in line with your navel.

Now relax your shoulders and turn your head to the right. Soften and widen the front edge of your thoracic diaphragm and turn from the back edge. To deepen the twist of your rib cage, turn the left side of your thoracic diaphragm toward the right side of your respiratory diaphragm, and lift the right side of your thoracic diaphragm away from the left side of your respiratory diaphragm. If the left side of your rib cage comes in contact with your right thigh, wrap your left arm around your right leg, and take hold of your right wrist behind your back.

Remain in Marichyasana III for another 30 seconds. Lengthen your left leg and turn, first, from the back edge of your pelvic diaphragm; then from the back edge of your respiratory diaphragm; and finally, from the back edge of your thoracic diaphragm. Coordinate the movement of the three diaphragms. Then release and repeat to the other side.

RELATED POSES. Bharadvajasana II, other sitting twists

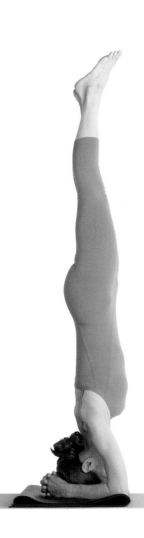

3.15
Salamba Sirsasana

SALAMBA SIRSASANA
HEADSTAND

PROPS
• set up as determined in Chapter 2

In Salamba Sirsasana (Figure 3.15), align your thoracic diaphragm parallel to the floor in order to balance your front rib cage and back rib cage.

Prepare for Salamba Sirsasana as described in Chapter 2. As you walk your feet in toward your head, lift the back edge of your pelvic diaphragm away from the back edge of your respiratory diaphragm. As you raise your legs, draw the center of your perineum into your body.

In Salamba Sirsasana, observe whether your thoracic diaphragm is tilted or parallel to the floor. If your thoracic diaphragm is tilted, the front edge is probably closer to the floor than the back edge, and your rib cage may be tilted as well. In this case, broaden the back edge of your thoracic diaphragm, and move it toward your shoulders; at the same time, lift the sides of your thoracic diaphragm away from your elbows. Feel how your rib cage and pelvis realign as you make this adjustment.

When your thoracic diaphragm is parallel to the floor, widen the back edge of your respiratory diaphragm, and lift your legs away from the sides of your respiratory diaphragm. Then broaden the back edge of your pelvic diaphragm, so that the center of your perineum is in line with the center of your respiratory diaphragm, and lift your legs away from the sides of your pelvic diaphragm.

Maintain this position for 3 to 5 minutes. Continue to widen your thoracic diaphragm and to lift the sides of your thoracic diaphragm away from your elbows. Check that all three diaphragms are parallel to the floor. When you are ready to come down, lift the back edge of your pelvic diaphragm away from the back edge of your respiratory diaphragm, and draw the center of your perineum into your body as you descend your legs. Rest in Adho Mukha Virasana (Child's Pose, Figure 3.11b).

RELATED POSES. Salamba Sirsasana variations

SALAMBA SARVANGASANA
SHOULDERSTAND

PROPS
• set up as determined in Chapter 1

In Salamba Sarvangasana (Figure 3.16), bring your thoracic diaphragm parallel to the floor to create a stable foundation for the pose.

Come into Salamba Sarvangasana as described in Chapter 1. First, widen your shoulders and lift the sides of your rib cage; then check whether your thoracic diaphragm is tilted or parallel to the floor. (If the back edge of your thoracic diaphragm

3.16
Salamba Sarvangasana

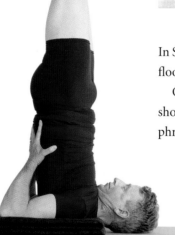

is closer to the floor than the front edge, the back of your body is dropping, rather than lifting.) To bring your thoracic diaphragm parallel to the floor, relax your shoulder blades and lift the back edge of your thoracic diaphragm away from the floor. At the same time, lengthen from the sides of your thoracic diaphragm toward your inner elbows, and turn the front edge of your thoracic diaphragm toward the base of your throat. As your thoracic diaphragm comes parallel to the floor, you will feel the back of your rib cage lift.

Then lift the back edge of your respiratory diaphragm away from the back edge of your thoracic diaphragm; simultaneously, lift your legs away from the sides of your respiratory diaphragm. Next, broaden the circumference of your pelvic diaphragm, and lift the back edge of your pelvic diaphragm away from the back edge of your respiratory diaphragm. Finally, lift your legs away from the sides of your pelvic diaphragm. Feel how your three diaphragms are suspended vertically one above another.

Remain in Salamba Sarvangasana for 3 to 10 minutes. Relax and widen your thoracic diaphragm. Lengthen from the sides of your thoracic diaphragm toward your inner elbows, and lift the back edge of your thoracic diaphragm away from the floor. Move the base of your skull away from the front edge of your thoracic diaphragm and soften your eyes. When you are ready to come into Halasana (Figure 3.17), lift the back edge of your pelvic diaphragm away from the back edge of your respiratory diaphragm to keep your lumbar spine long; then draw the center of your perineum into your body as you descend your legs

RELATED POSES. Setu Bandhasana

HALASANA
PLOUGH POSE

PROPS
• set up as determined in Chapter 1

In Halasana (Figure 3.17), your pelvis is aligned over your neck, rather than over your shoulders, to lengthen your lumbar spine and lift the back of your rib cage.

Come into Halasana from Salamba Sarvangasana as described for Figure 3.16. Relax your shoulder girdle and lift the back edge of your thoracic diaphragm away from the floor. At the same time, lengthen from the sides of your thoracic diaphragm toward your inner elbows, and turn the front edge of your thoracic diaphragm toward the base of your throat, so that your thoracic diaphragm is parallel to the floor.

Then lift the back edge of your respiratory diaphragm away from the back edge of your thoracic diaphragm to release your rib cage. Now lift the back edge of your pelvic diaphragm away from the back edge of your respiratory diaphragm to lengthen your

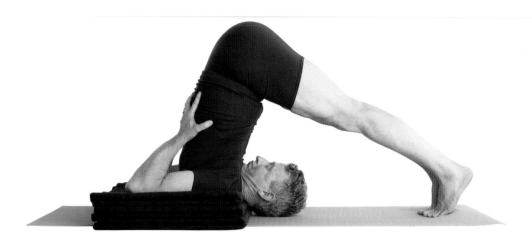

3.17
Halasana

lumbar spine; at the same time, lengthen your legs from the sides of your pelvic diaphragm. Repeat these instructions two or three times, until the back of your body feels fully lifted.

Remain in Halasana for one-third to one-half the time you spent in Salamba Sarvangasana. Relax and widen your thoracic diaphragm. Release the base of your skull away from the front edge of your thoracic diaphragm, and draw your eyes deeper into their sockets. When you have reached a place of stillness, roll out of the pose, and rest with your shoulders off the folded edge of your blankets.

PASCHIMOTTANASANA WITH HANDS ON BLOCKS
SITTING FORWARD BEND

PROPS
- 1 nonskid mat
- 1 blanket or wedge
- 2 blocks

In Paschimottanasana with Hands on Blocks (Figure 3.18), bring your pelvic diaphragm parallel to the floor to create space in your hip joints and deepen your forward bend.

Place a folded blanket or wedge on your mat. Then sit with your sitting bones on the edge of the blanket or wedge, and your legs extended. Place a block to the outside of each foot to support your hands. (If you are more flexible, lay the blocks flat. If you are less flexible, stand them on end.) With an inhalation, raise your arms overhead. With an exhalation, lift your rib cage away from the back edge of your respiratory diaphragm as you extend your torso over your thighs. Place your hands on the blocks with your palms flat. (Adjust the position of the blocks, if necessary, so that your arms are fully extended.)

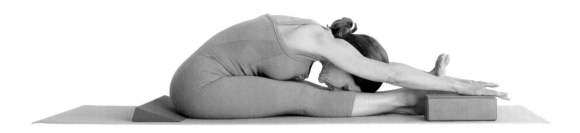

3.18

Paschimottanasana with Hands on Blocks

In Paschimottanasana with Hands on Blocks, move the back edge of your pelvic diaphragm away from the back edge of your respiratory diaphragm to lengthen your lumbar spine. Then move the back edge of your respiratory diaphragm toward the back edge of your thoracic diaphragm to release your thoracic spine. Finally, soften and widen the back edge of your thoracic diaphragm, and move it toward your shoulders to release your cervical spine.

When the back of your body is fully extended, bring your awareness to the front of your body. Draw your groins deeper into your body, and lengthen the sides of your pelvic diaphragm away from your groins. Then gently turn your xiphoid process toward your navel, widen your midsternum, and turn the front edge of your thoracic diaphragm away from the base of your throat. Feel how the front of your brain relaxes with this movement.

Remain in this position for 1 to 2 minutes, allowing your front body to rest on your back body. To come out of the pose, extend your arms overhead and lift your torso with an inhalation. With an exhalation, turn your palms out and lower your arms to your sides.

JANU SIRSASANA WITH HANDS ON BLOCKS
HEAD—OF—THE—KNEE POSE

PROPS
- 1 nonskid mat
- 2 blocks
- 1 blanket or wedge

This variation of Janu Sirsasana with Hands on Blocks (Figure 3.19) focuses on lengthening both sides of the torso evenly.

Place a folded blanket or wedge on your mat. Then sit with your sitting bones on the edge of the blanket or wedge and your legs extended. Bend your right knee and place your right heel near your right groin, with the top of your foot on the floor. Place a block on either side of your left foot to support your hands. (If you are more flexible, lay the blocks flat. If you are less flexible, stand them on end.)

With an inhalation, raise your arms overhead and turn your sternum to face your left foot. With an exhalation, lift your rib cage away from the back edge of your respiratory diaphragm as you lengthen your torso over your left leg. Place your hands on the blocks with your palms flat. (Adjust the position of the blocks, if necessary, so that your arms are fully extended.)

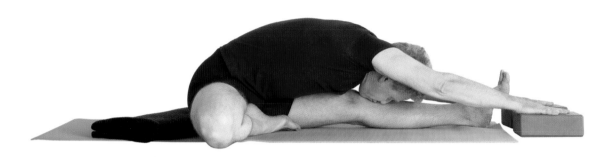

3.19

Janu Sirsasana with Hands on Blocks

In Janu Sirsasana with Hands on Blocks, widen your pelvic diaphragm toward your bent leg, as you shift your respiratory diaphragm over the thigh of your extended leg. Draw the left side of your pelvic diaphragm away from your left leg, and lift the left side of your respiratory diaphragm to lengthen the left side of your waist. Then relax your shoulders and lift the left side of your thoracic diaphragm away from the left side of your respiratory diaphragm to lengthen the left side of your rib cage. Broaden the back edge of your thoracic diaphragm, and turn the front edge away from the base of your throat to release your head and neck.

Remain in Janu Sirsasana with Hands on Blocks for 1 minute. Draw your left groin into your body, and widen the back edge of your pelvic diaphragm. Turn your xiphoid process gently toward your navel, and widen the back edge of your respiratory diaphragm. Then broaden the back edge of your thoracic diaphragm, and turn the front edge away from the base of your throat to release your head and neck.

To come out of the pose, extend your arms overhead and lift your torso with an inhalation. Then turn your palms out, and lower your arms with an exhalation.

RELATED POSES. Other sitting forward bends

UJJAYI PRANAYAMA RESTING
BASIC YOGA BREATHING

PROPS
- 1 nonskid mat
- 1 bolster

OPTIONAL PROPS
- 2 or 3 blankets

This variation of Ujjayi Pranayama Resting, practiced in Adho Mukha Virasana with a Bolster (Figure 3.20), focuses on the movement of the pelvic diaphragm.

Sit on your heels on a nonskid mat with your knees body-width apart, and place a bolster lengthwise between your thighs. (If you do not have a bolster, use two or three blankets folded in half lengthwise, and stack them one on top of the other.) Rest the front of your torso on the bolster, with your arms overhead and your head turned to one side. If your shoulders are not higher than your pelvis, add another blanket under your rib cage.

3.20
Adho Mukha Virasana with a Bolster

Once you are settled comfortably in Adho Mukha Virasana with a Bolster, relax your shoulders and arms, and focus on your lower abdomen. With a deep, soft inhalation, broaden your pelvic diaphragm. Start from the back edge of your pelvic diaphragm, where it is tightest, and let the movement gradually expand. With each exhalation, release your inner groins and the muscles of your lower back. Synchronize the movement of your breath with the movement of your pelvic diaphragm, so that body and breath become one. Continue this cycle for 2 to 3 minutes. Then turn your head to the other side, and repeat for an equal length of time.

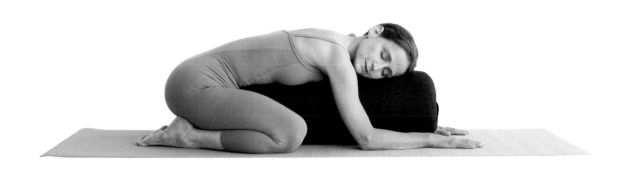

UJJAYI PRANAYAMA SITTING
BASIC YOGA BREATHING

PROPS	OPTIONAL PROPS
• 1 nonskid mat	• 1 or 2 blocks or blankets
• 1 blanket	• 1 wedge

This variation of Ujjayi Pranayama Sitting develops awareness and movement of the three diaphragms.

Rest in Savasana (Figure 3.22) for 2 or 3 minutes before you begin your breathing practice. Then sit on your mat at the edge of a folded blanket in your most comfortable sitting position: Padmasana (Lotus Pose, Figure 3.21), Siddhasana (Perfect Pose, Figure 4.23), Sukhasana (Easy Pose, Figure 6.22), or Virasana (Hero Pose, Figure 5.24). If your knees are not in contact with the floor, use blocks or blankets to support them. (You can also use a wedge under your sitting bones to give an additional lift to your pelvis and spine.) Then bring your elbows to the sides of your waist, and place your hands on your thighs. Close your eyes gently and drop your chin to your sternal notch. Broaden your shoulders and release the base of your neck without collapsing your spine.

Phase 1. Begin with a deep, soft exhalation. With a deep inhalation, widen the back edge of your pelvic diaphragm, and lift the center of your perineum into your body. At the same time, lift your lumbar spine and the sides of your rib cage. With an exhalation, maintain the lift of your torso, as your lower abdominal muscles are drawn

3.21
Padmasana

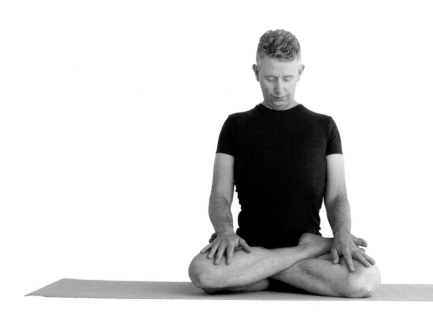

back toward the center of your perineum. Repeat this cycle for 2 to 3 minutes, and then change the cross of your legs.

Phase 2. Begin with a deep, soft exhalation. With each inhalation, widen the back edge of your respiratory diaphragm, and lift from the sides of your respiratory diaphragm. Keep the sides of your respiratory diaphragm parallel to the floor throughout your inhalation, so that the front corners do not lift higher than the back corners. Let your midsternum broaden. With the exhalation, let your nasal bones narrow, and release your breath slowly through the channel of your upper nostrils. Repeat this cycle for 2 to 3 minutes, and then change the cross of your legs.

Phase 3. Begin with a deep, soft exhalation. With a deep inhalation, widen the back edge of your thoracic diaphragm, and release the base of your neck. At the same time, draw the sides of your thoracic diaphragm gently back and down to stabilize your shoulders, but lift the front edge of your thoracic diaphragm toward the base of your throat. Let the breath move softly into your upper lungs. With the exhalation, keep your thoracic diaphragm broad, and clear the breath from your sinus cavities. Repeat this cycle for 2 to 3 minutes, and then change the cross of your legs.

Phase 4. Finally, try to synchronize the movement of all three diaphragms. Begin with a deep, soft exhalation. With a deep inhalation, widen the back edge of your pelvic diaphragm, and lift from the center of your perineum. As you lift from the center of your perineum, widen the back edge of your respiratory diaphragm, and lift your rib cage from the sides of your respiratory diaphragm. As you lift from the sides of your respiratory diaphragm, widen the back edge of your thoracic diaphragm, and lift the front edge toward the base of your throat. When you coordinate the movement of your three diaphragms in this way, you will find that your inhalation grows softer and deeper, and requires less effort. Throughout the exhalation, maintain the balance of your three diaphragms and the lift of your spine. Repeat this cycle for 2 to 3 minutes.

When you are finished, rest in Savasana.

SAVASANA
RELAXATION POSE

PROP
• 1 nonskid mat

OPTIONAL PROP
• 1 blanket

In this variation of Savasana (Figure 3.22), observe the movement of your respiratory diaphragm with each cycle of breath.

Lie on your back on a nonskid mat with your knees bent and your feet on the floor in line with your sitting bones. (If the base of your skull feels tight, place a folded blanket under your head and neck.) Bend your elbows and press the back of your upper arms into the floor. Keep equal weight on your inner and outer elbows as you straighten your arms and rest the back of your hands on the floor. Then press your sacrum into the floor, and extend your legs, one at a time. Relax your pelvis and knees, and allow your legs to roll out.

Close your eyes and soften your inward gaze. With each inhalation, observe the expansion of your respiratory diaphragm. With each exhalation, follow the movement of your breath down the front of your lumbar spine. Continue in Savasana for 5 to 10 minutes. As your breathing becomes deeper and softer, you will enter a place of stillness, a quiet pause at the end of exhalation.

When you feel rested, bend your knees and turn onto your side before sitting up. Namaste.

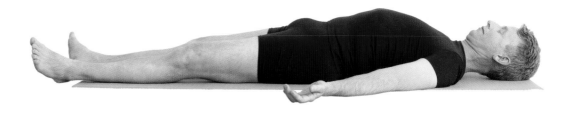

► PRACTICE SEQUENCE

Tadasana

Adho Mukha Svanasana

Utthita Parsvakonasana

Padangusthasana

Uttanasana

Ardha Chandrasana

Parivrtta Ardha Chandrasana at the Wall

Virabhadrasana I

Adho Mukha Vrksasana at the Wall

Ustrasana

Urdhva Dhanurasana

Marichyasana III

Salamba Sirsasana

Salamba Sarvangasana

Halasana

Paschimottanasana with Hands on Blocks

Janu Sirsasana with Hands on Blocks

Ujjayi Pranayama Resting

Ujjayi Pranayama Sitting

Savasana

4 BALANCE YOUR STERNUM

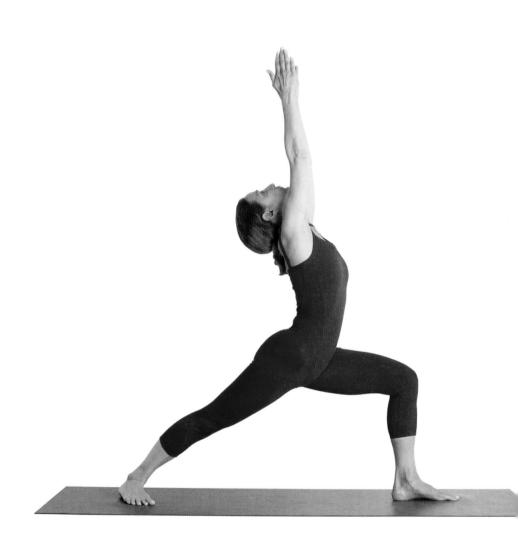

ONE OF B. K. S. IYENGAR'S most profound insights into the language of the body is that the sternum, or breastbone, is the key to opening the chest. For generations, Iyengar students have been instructed to "lift the sternum," and yet for a long time I misinterpreted this instruction, because I did not fully understand the anatomy, or composite nature, of the sternum. In recent years, I sensed in my own practice that the upper sternum should move in a different direction from the mid-sternum, but it wasn't until a chiropractor friend placed in my hand, like sacred relics, a small, medallion-shaped manubrium together with a long sternal body, that I realized what I had intuited through yoga was anatomically possible.

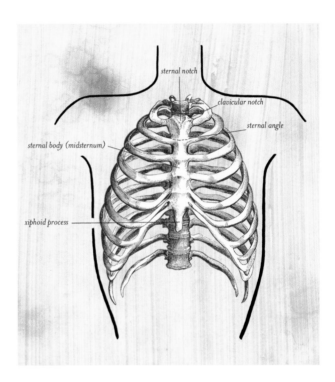

The sternum (which means "chest," or "breast") is a long, flat bone that extends from the notch at the base of the throat down the midline of the front body to the notch at the base of the rib cage. Shaped like a dagger pointing downward, the sternum is composed of three parts: the manubrium, or upper sternum; the sternal body (which I refer to as the midsternum); and the xiphoid process (Figure 4.1).

The manubrium, or upper sternum, is wider than the sternal body, and takes its name from the Latin word meaning "handle." At the center of the upper edge of the manubrium is a notch called the sternal, or jugular, notch. Along the side edges of the manubrium are other sets of notches, where the collarbones and first ribs articulate with the manubrium. The lower edge of the manubrium and the upper edge of the sternal body form a cartilaginous joint called the sternal angle, which, for most individuals, becomes fused by adulthood.

The sternal body (midsternum) develops from four separate centers that gradually ossify and fuse together, leaving three transverse ridges on the anterior, or front, surface of the bone as vestiges of this process. Notice how the ribs articulate with the sternum at the level of these junctures. The second ribs articulate at the sternal angle; the third, fourth, and fifth ribs at the level of the three transverse ridges; and the sixth and seventh ribs at the juncture between the sternal body and the xiphoid process.

The xiphoid protrudes from the base of the sternal body, and is the tip of the dagger. *Xiphoid* comes from a Greek word meaning "sword shaped." In children, the xiphoid process consists of hyaline cartilage, which does not ossify completely until about the age of forty. The xiphoid process is intimately linked with our breathing, and thus important energetically, because a major portion of the diaphragm originates here.

In form and function, the sternum bears a striking resemblance to the sacrum. The

4.1
Sternum and Rib Cage (front view)

fusion of the sternal body is similar to the fusion of the five vertebrae that form the sacrum, along with its four transverse ridges. The xiphoid process is like the tail of the sternum, just as the coccyx is the tail of the sacrum. Any movement of the xiphoid process directly affects the tone and quality of the respiratory diaphragm, just as the coccyx affects the pelvic diaphragm.

The sacrum is a vital center of communication linking the legs, pelvis, and lumbar spine. If your sacrum is tilted to the right or left, or if your sacrum is too deep or too near the surface of the body, then your hip joints, sacroiliac joints, and lumbar spine will be more vulnerable to injury.

In a similar way, the manubrium, or upper sternum, is the center of communication, or control panel, for the arms, shoulder girdle, and rib cage. If your manubrium is tilted to the right or left, or if your manubrium is too deep or too prominent, your shoulder girdle, shoulder joints, and, ultimately, your cervical spine will be adversely affected.

Take a moment to check in the mirror whether your manubrium is facing directly forward. If your manubrium is tilted to the right or left, it may be the result of a serious fall, a car accident, or a sudden impact to your shoulder. When your manubrium is torqued or displaced for any reason, your whole shoulder girdle is forced out of alignment, with one shoulder thrown forward and the other one back. In this case, you may experience a shoulder imbalance in Adho Mukha Svanasana (Figure 4.6), Adho Mukha Vrksasana at the Wall (Figure 3.11a), and Salamba Sirsasana (Figure 4.17); yet the remedy lies not in adjusting your shoulders, but in aligning your manubrium with the frontal plane of your body.

If your manubrium is too deep or too prominent, it is usually the result of long-term postural habits. If you tend to slouch or hunch your shoulders, then your manubrium sinks down, your upper back rounds, and your head is thrown forward, thus shortening the back of your neck. In this situation, where your neck is chronically overarched, you are especially prone to neck injuries in Salamba Sirsasana.

On the other hand, if you push your manubrium forward in military style to open your chest, your thoracic spine tends to flatten, and you lose the natural curve of your neck. When the curve of your neck is flattened or, in extreme cases, reversed, you are much more vulnerable to neck injuries in Salamba Sarvangasana (Figure 4.18).

When you hear the instruction in a yoga class, "Lift your sternum," remember the distinction between your manubrium and your sternal body. If you lift from your manubrium, you will force the upper sternum out of your body and grip your upper spine. Instead, bring your awareness to your heart center, and broaden and lift from your midsternum, so that your manubrium turns upward and rests back into your body (Figure 4.2).

The position of your manubrium is greatly affected by the muscles that fill the hollow space between your collarbones and your upper ribs on either side of your

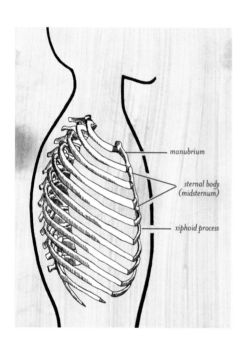

4.2
Sternum and Rib Cage (side view)

manubrium

sternal body (midsternum)

xiphoid process

manubrium. B. K. S. Iyengar calls these indentations "the eyes of the chest," because they feel like sockets and act like the eyes (Figure 4.3). When you relax the tension in your eyes, notice how your eyeballs draw back into your eye sockets, filling them more completely. When you make this adjustment, even the position of your head changes: your chin drops slightly and the tightness at the base of your skull releases.

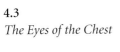

4.3
The Eyes of the Chest

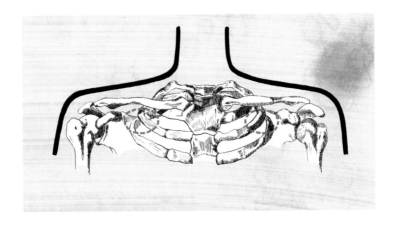

In the same way, drawing the eyes of your chest back into your body releases tension in your shoulder girdle, and allows your manubrium to rest in its natural place. When your pectoral muscles are tight, your shoulders are pulled forward, your manubrium collapses, and the eyes of your chest feel shallow and closed. Drawing the eyes of your chest back into your body involves releasing the superficial pectoral muscles, and contacting the muscles that lie deeper in the sockets. When this happens, you feel a depth and fullness in the eyes of the chest, and your manubrium is soft and broad.

The third part of the sternum, the xiphoid process, plays a special role in coordinating the action of the sternum and the spine. Because the diaphragm connects the xiphoid process and the first lumbar vertebra, any movement of the xiphoid directly affects the lumbar-thoracic joint, the vital hinge between the lumbar and the thoracic spine. In this way, the xiphoid process both signals and reflects the direction of the spine. In backbends, the xiphoid process lifts away from the sides of the navel to allow for maximum extension of the spine. In forward bends, the xiphoid process turns toward the sides of the navel to allow for the full release of the spine.

In this chapter, we practice leading neither from the upper sternum nor from the xiphoid process, but from the midsternum, or heart area. When you lead from the upper sternum, you overwork and overflatten your upper spine. When you lead from the xiphoid process, you overwork and overarch your lumbar spine. When your sternum is balanced, your midsternum leads (is most prominent), and your whole spine lengthens harmoniously. A balanced sternum reflects a balanced spine.

The poses in the following sequence develop your awareness of the three parts of the sternum—the manubrium, midsternum, and xiphoid process—and help bring them into balance.

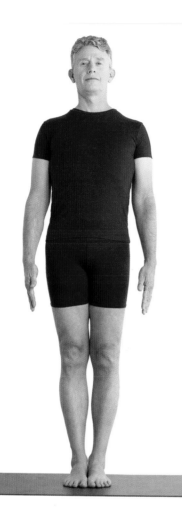

TADASANA
MOUNTAIN POSE

PROP

• 1 nonskid mat

In Tadasana (Figure 4.4), the sternum is like the shaft of a bow: the center, or midsternum, moves forward and the ends are drawn back to give strength and resilience to the thoracic spine.

Stand on your mat in Tadasana with your feet together and your arms by the sides of your body. Adjust your pelvis so that the center of your perineum is directly in line with the center of your respiratory diaphragm. From the sides of your pelvic diaphragm, lengthen down through your inner legs; from the center of your perineum, lift your spine. Widen your shoulders and lift from the sides of your chest.

4.4
Tadasana

Now bring your awareness to your heart center. Let your midsternum broaden and lift, so that it comes level with your front rib cage. At the same time, widen and lift your xiphoid process away from the sides of your navel. Draw the eyes of your chest deeper into their sockets, and let your manubrium turn gently toward your head. Maintain this position for several breaths, allowing your midsternum to lead you in the pose. Feel your heart center become quiet yet physically alert. Return to Tadasana after each of the standing poses.

facing page:
4.5
Tadasana with a Partner

TADASANA WITH A PARTNER
MOUNTAIN POSE

PROP

• 1 nonskid mat

This variation of Tadasana with a Partner (Figure 4.5) helps you evaluate the alignment of your manubrium and understand its relationship with your upper thoracic spine.

When you are the helper, let your partner stand on her mat in Tadasana with her feet together and her spine fully lengthened. Place the palm of one hand on your partner's manubrium, and the palm of your other hand on her upper thoracic spine.

If your partner's manubrium presses into your hand at the front of the body, but her thoracic spine drops away from your hand at the back of the body, your partner's manubrium is overly prominent, and her upper thoracic spine may be somewhat flattened.

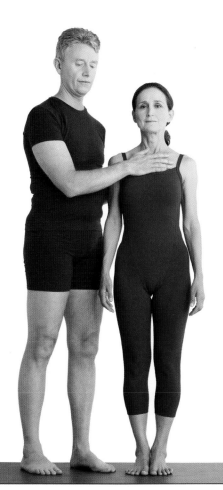

If your partner's manubrium sinks away from your hand at the front of the body, but her thoracic spine presses into your hand at the back of the body, your partner's manubrium is collapsed, and her upper thoracic spine may be overly rounded.

Encourage your partner to adjust her pose so that her manubrium rests lightly against the palm of one hand and her upper thoracic spine fills the palm of your other hand. Her front body and back body will then be in dynamic balance, moving gently away from each other.

Occasionally, you will find a partner or student whose manubrium collapses at the front of the body, but whose upper thoracic is overly flattened at the back of the body. Your hands will feel as though they are moving toward each other, rather than away from each other. In this case, your partner probably has a very wide, shallow, boxlike rib cage. (See Chapter 6 for a description of the basic shapes of the ribcage.)

When you have finished, change roles with your partner.

ADHO MUKHA SVANASANA
DOWNWARD-FACING DOG POSE

PROP

- 1 nonskid mat

In this variation of Adho Mukha Svanasana (Figure 4.6), proper alignment of the sternum helps to balance the shoulders and lengthen the spine.

Start in a kneeling position on your mat, with your wrists in line with your shoulders and your pelvis over your knees. As you lengthen down through your arms, draw the eyes of your chest deeper into their sockets, and allow your upper back to round. Then turn your toes under, lift your pelvis, and straighten your legs. At the same time, firm your inner elbows and lengthen the sides of your chest away from your inner arms.

In Adho Mukha Svanasana, first check that your manubrium is properly aligned with the frontal plane of your body. If your manubrium turns to the right or left, your shoulders are imbalanced. In this case, turn your manubrium so that it faces directly forward, and feel the corresponding release in your shoulder joints. Then check the alignment of your midsternum. If your midsternum turns to the right or left, your rib cage is torqued. In this event, stabilize your manubrium and gently bring your midsternum into the frontal plane, as you continue to lengthen your spine.

To release your thoracic spine, lift your rib cage away from the eyes of your chest, and lengthen the sides of your chest. To release and lengthen your lumbar spine, turn

4.6
Adho Mukha Svanasana

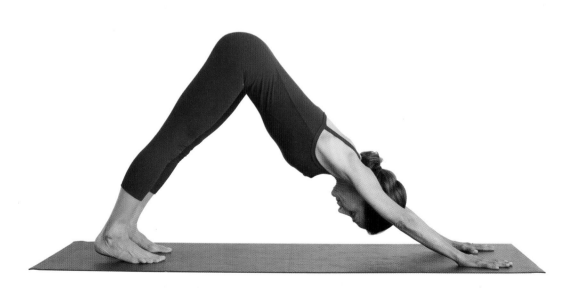

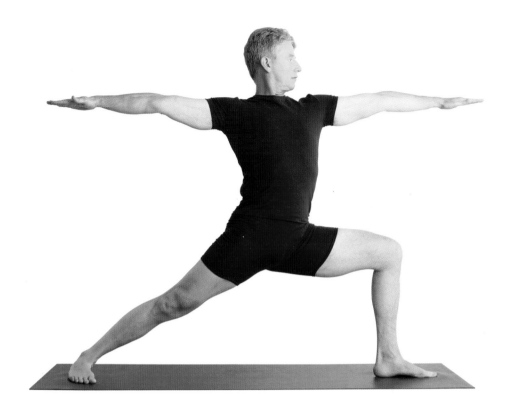

4.7
Virabhadrasana II

your xiphoid process toward your navel, and lengthen the sides of your navel toward your inner groins. Finally, broaden your midsternum, so that your whole rib cage expands. Maintain this position for another minute, turning your xiphoid process toward your navel, broadening your midsternum, and lengthening your spine. Then bend your knees and rest in Adho Mukha Virasana (Child's Pose, Figure 3.11b).

Practice Notes. When you are in Adho Mukha Svanasana, which part of your sternum is leading, or most prominent: your manubrium, midsternum, or xiphoid process? If your manubrium leads, you are overworking your shoulders and sinking into your shoulder joints. In this case, let your manubrium rest back into your body, and soften the eyes of your chest. If your xiphoid process is most prominent, your lower ribs are protruding and your lumbar spine is dropping. In this case, turn and lift your xiphoid process toward your navel, and bring your midsternum toward the surface of your body. When your midsternum leads, you can lift your rib cage away from your shoulder joints and achieve maximum length in your spine.

VIRABHADRASANA II
WARRIOR POSE II

PROP
• 1 nonskid mat

In this variation of Virabhadrasana II (Figure 4.7), ideally, your sternum will be vertically aligned, so that you lead with your midsternum, not with your xiphoid process or manubrium.

Stand on your mat in Tadasana (Figure 4.4), and separate your feet about 4 to 4½ feet apart. Turn your right foot out 90 degrees and your left foot in 30 degrees. Bring the center of your perineum directly in line with the center of your respiratory diaphragm. With an inhalation, broaden your midsternum and raise your arms out to the side to shoulder level. With an exhalation, lengthen from your xiphoid process to your inner left leg, as you bend your right knee to form a right angle. Turn your head to look over your right hand.

In Virabhadrasana II, widen the back edge of your respiratory diaphragm, and lengthen from your xiphoid process to your inner left leg. At the same time, widen your midsternum and turn it to face directly forward. Soften the eyes of your chest, and draw them deeper into your body. Then let your manubrium turn toward your head and rest back into your body, as you extend your arms away from your upper thoracic spine. Maintain this position for several breaths; then repeat to the other side.

RELATED POSES. Utthita Trikonasana, Utthita Parsvakonasana, Ardha Chandrasana

PADANGUSTHASANA
TOE-HOLDING POSE

PROP
• 1 nonskid mat

OPTIONAL PROP
• 1 block

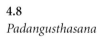

4.8
Padangusthasana

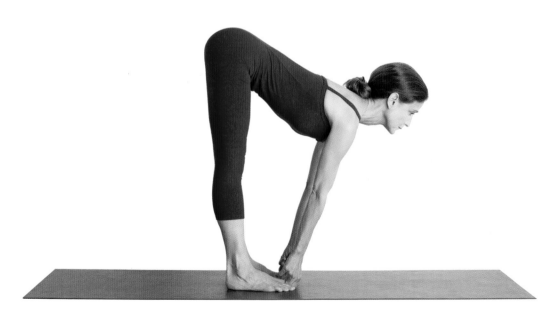

In this variation of Padangusthasana (Figure 4.8), the xiphoid process lifts away from the sides of the navel to arch and extend the spine.

Stand on your mat in Tadasana (Figure 4.4) with your feet a few inches apart, and place your hands on your hips. With an inhalation, lift the sides of your rib cage away from the back edge of your respiratory diaphragm. At the same time, lift your xiphoid process away from the sides of your navel and broaden your midsternum. Then turn your manubrium toward your head, and let your head drop back. With an exhalation, draw your groins up into your body, and lengthen your torso forward, leading with your midsternum, not your xiphoid process. When your torso is parallel to the floor, extend your arms and wrap your second and third fingers around your big toes. (If you cannot take hold of your toes without rounding your back, place a block directly in front of your feet to support your hands.)

In Padangusthasana, keep the back edge of your respiratory diaphragm broad, and lengthen your lumbar spine away from your sacrum. Lift your xiphoid process away from the sides of your navel to release your thoracic spine. Turn your manubrium toward your head to release your cervical spine. Then broaden your midsternum to release your shoulders, and lengthen through the crown of your head. Maintain this position for several breaths; then return to Tadasana.

RELATED POSE. Prasarita Padottanasana (Phase 1)

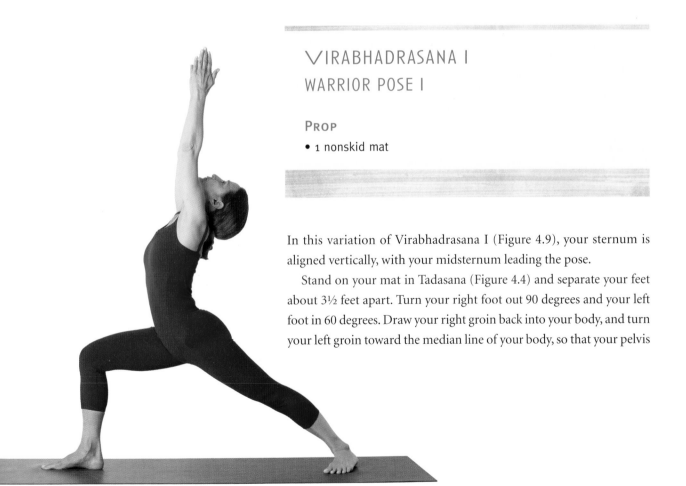

4.9
Virabhadrasana I

VIRABHADRASANA I
WARRIOR POSE I

PROP
• 1 nonskid mat

In this variation of Virabhadrasana I (Figure 4.9), your sternum is aligned vertically, with your midsternum leading the pose.

Stand on your mat in Tadasana (Figure 4.4) and separate your feet about 3½ feet apart. Turn your right foot out 90 degrees and your left foot in 60 degrees. Draw your right groin back into your body, and turn your left groin toward the median line of your body, so that your pelvis directly faces your right leg. Then place your hands on your hips with your thumbs pressing down at the top edge of your sacrum. Broaden the back edge of your respiratory diaphragm, and lift from the sides of your chest. At the same time, lift your xiphoid process away from the sides of your navel, and lengthen down through your inner left leg. With an inhalation, broaden and lift your midsternum as you raise your arms overhead. With an exhalation, bend your right knee without dropping your xiphoid process.

In Virabhadrasana I, continue to lift your xiphoid process away from the sides of your navel, and lengthen down through your inner left leg. Soften and broaden your midsternum so that it lifts to the level of your front rib cage and turns gently toward the ceiling. Check that your midsternum is leading you into the pose, not your xiphoid process. Then turn your manubrium toward your head, and let it rest back into your body. Feel how your cervical spine releases and your head drops back more easily. Maintain this position for 30 seconds more; then lift out of the pose, and repeat to the other side.

Practice Notes. Ideally, in Virabhadrasana I, your xiphoid process will be aligned directly over your navel. If your xiphoid process is forward of your navel, your pelvis is tilted forward too much and your lumbar spine is overarched. If your navel is forward of your xiphoid process, you may be pulling your shoulder girdle back too far or overtucking your pelvis. To avoid compression of your lumbar spine in Virabhadrasana I, bring your shoulder joints directly over your hip joints and your xiphoid process in line with your navel.

4.10
Uttanasana

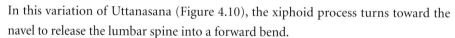

UTTANASANA
STANDING FORWARD BEND

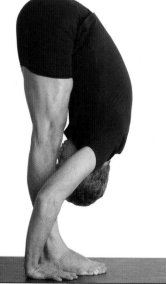

PROP
• 1 nonskid mat

OPTIONAL PROP
• 1 block

In this variation of Uttanasana (Figure 4.10), the xiphoid process turns toward the navel to release the lumbar spine into a forward bend.

Stand in Tadasana (Figure 4.4) with your feet a few inches apart, and place your hands on your hips. With an inhalation, bring the center of your perineum directly in line with the center of your respiratory diaphragm. With an exhalation, draw your groins up into your body and lengthen your torso forward, leading with your midsternum—not your xiphoid process—so that your spine maintains a neutral position. When your pelvis has rotated to its maximum, place your hands on the floor by the sides of your feet with your fingers facing forward, so that your upper arms are parallel to each other. (If you cannot reach the floor easily, use a block placed in front of your feet to support your hands.)

In Uttanasana, turn your xiphoid process toward your navel to release your lumbar spine and lengthen your kidneys. Then widen your midthoracic vertebrae, and bring your midsternum toward your thighs. Soften the eyes of your chest, and lengthen toward your inner elbows from deep in the sockets. Let your manubrium rest back into your body, and release the base of your skull, so that your head hangs freely. Maintain this position for another minute; then place your hands on your hips, lengthen through the crown of your head, and return to Tadasana with a neutral spine.

Related Pose. Prasarita Padottanasana (Phase 2)

4.11
Parivrtta Trikonasana

PARIVRTTA TRIKONASANA
REVOLVED TRIANGLE POSE

PROP
• 1 nonskid mat

OPTIONAL PROP
• 1 block

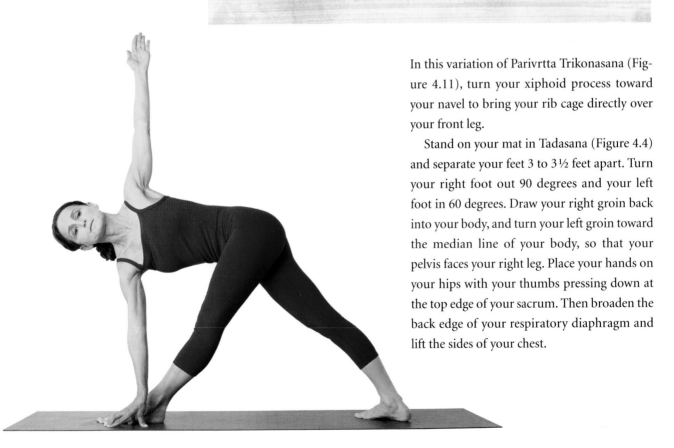

In this variation of Parivrtta Trikonasana (Figure 4.11), turn your xiphoid process toward your navel to bring your rib cage directly over your front leg.

Stand on your mat in Tadasana (Figure 4.4) and separate your feet 3 to 3½ feet apart. Turn your right foot out 90 degrees and your left foot in 60 degrees. Draw your right groin back into your body, and turn your left groin toward the median line of your body, so that your pelvis faces your right leg. Place your hands on your hips with your thumbs pressing down at the top edge of your sacrum. Then broaden the back edge of your respiratory diaphragm and lift the sides of your chest.

With an inhalation, raise your left arm overhead, and turn your midsternum to face your right leg. With an exhalation, move your xiphoid process toward the sides of your navel as you extend your torso over your right leg. When your spine is parallel to the floor, place your left hand on the floor directly below your left shoulder, either at your inner ankle or your outer ankle, depending on your flexibility. (Use a block under your hand, if necessary.) Then bring the crown of your head in line with the center of your perineum, and raise your right arm toward the ceiling.

In Parivrtta Trikonasana, continue to move your xiphoid process toward the sides of your navel to bring your shoulder girdle over your front leg. At the same time, broaden your midsternum so that it rises to the level of your front rib cage and deepens your twist. Check that your midsternum leads you into the pose, not your xiphoid process or manubrium. Let your manubrium turn gently toward your head to release and lengthen your cervical spine. Then soften the eyes of your chest, and lengthen your upper arms away from your upper thoracic spine. Maintain this position for several breaths, then repeat to the other side.

RELATED POSE. Parivrtta Ardha Chandrasana

URDHVA MUKHA SVANASANA
UPWARD-FACING DOG POSE

PROPS
- 1 nonskid mat
- 1 blanket

OPTIONAL PROP
- 2 blocks

In this variation of Urdhva Mukha Svanasana (Figure 4.12), the sternum is aligned vertically to avoid compression in the lumbar spine and open the chest.

Lie face down on your mat with your pelvis supported by a folded blanket and your legs extended. Then bend your elbows and place the palms of your hands on the floor by the sides of your waist, so that your upper arms are parallel. (If your arms are short in proportion to the length of your spine, use blocks under your hands to help lift your chest.) With an inhalation, lengthen the back of your arms toward your elbows and lift your head. With an exhalation, widen your midsternum and lift your rib cage away from your inner elbows as you straighten your arms.

In Urdhva Mukha Svanasana, lengthen your inner legs away from the sides of your navel; at the same time, lift your xiphoid process away from the sides of your navel. Then broaden your midsternum, lift the sides of your rib cage, and lengthen the back of your arms. Turn your manubrium toward your head, and draw the eyes of your chest deeper into their sockets. You can let your head drop back, but only if it feels comfortable for your neck.

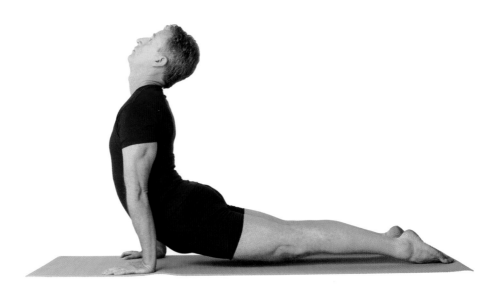

4.12
Urdhva Mukha Svanasana

Hold this position for several breaths. Lengthen your inner legs away from the sides of your navel. Lift your xiphoid process, broaden your midsternum, and turn your manubrium toward your head. Let your midsternum lead you in the pose. Feel the release in your cervical spine when your sternum is balanced. To come out of the pose, keep your upper arms parallel as you slowly bend your elbows; then rest with your forehead on the floor.

Practice Notes. When your sternum is properly balanced in Urdhva Mukha Svanasana, your xiphoid process is lifted without protruding forward; your midsternum faces directly forward and leads you in the pose; and your manubrium turns toward your head and rests back into your body. If your xiphoid process protrudes, your lumbar spine is overarched, and you may feel compression in your lumbar spine. If your manubrium protrudes, you are gripping your upper thoracic spine, and may feel discomfort in your shoulders or neck. Ideally, your sternum is vertically aligned in Urdhva Mukha Svanasana as in Tadasana (Figure 4.4).

USTRASANA
CAMEL POSE

PROPS
- 1 nonskid mat
- 1 blanket

OPTIONAL PROPS
- 3 blocks

This variation of Ustrasana (Figure 4.13) focuses on balancing the sternum to release the upper spine and avoid discomfort in the neck.

Place a folded blanket on top of your mat to protect your knees. Then kneel on the blanket with your feet hip-width apart. (If your feet have a tendency to slide together, place a block lengthwise between them to keep them stable.) Place your hands on your pelvis with your thumbs pressing down on the top edge of your sacrum, and lift the back edge of your respiratory diaphragm away from your sacrum. With an inhalation, lengthen your front thighs away from the sides of your navel; at the same time, lift your xiphoid process away from the sides of your navel. With an exhalation, broaden your midsternum and turn it to face the ceiling, as you let your head drop back, placing your hands on your heels with your arms extended. (If you have a neck injury or experience discomfort in your neck, keep your chin tucked into your chest or work with a partner supporting the weight of your head. If you cannot easily reach your heels, use blocks under your hands.)

In Ustrasana, lift your xiphoid process away from the sides of your navel. Lengthen the back of your arms and broaden your midsternum, so that it lifts gently to the level of your front rib cage. Let the eyes of your chest sink deeper into your body, and turn your manubrium toward your head. Release the base of your skull away from your manubrium and soften your eyes.

Maintain this position for several breaths, lifting your xiphoid process, broadening your midsternum, and drawing the eyes of your chest deeper into your body. To come out of the pose, place your hands on your sacrum, lift from your midsternum to return to a kneeling position, and sit back on your heels.

Practice Notes. When your sternum is balanced in Ustrasana, your xiphoid process is lifted without protruding; your midsternum faces directly toward the ceiling and forms the apex of the pose; and your manubrium rests back into your body. If your xiphoid process protrudes, you are collapsing and compressing your lumbar spine. If your manubrium is higher and more prominent than your midsternum, you will have difficulty releasing your head and neck.

4.13

Ustrasana

RELATED POSES. Salabhasana, Setu Bandhasana, other backbends

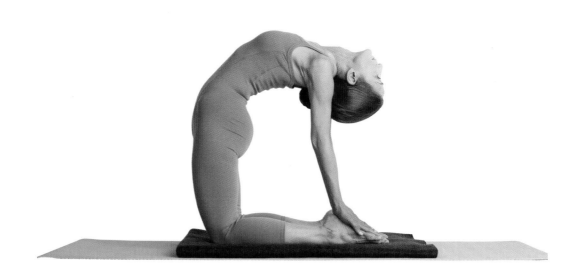

Urdhva Dhanurasana
Upward-Facing Bow Pose

Prop	Optional Props	
• 1 nonskid mat	• 2 blocks	• 1 wall
	• 1 wedge	• 1 strap

In this variation of Urdhva Dhanurasana (Figure 4.14), your manubrium turns to face the floor, and your midsternum feels vertically aligned.

Lie on your back with your arms extended overhead. Bend your knees and place your feet flat on the floor in line with your sitting bones and parallel to each other. Bend your elbows and place the palms of your hands flat on the floor on either side of your head, so that your upper arms are parallel to each other. With an inhalation, lengthen the sides of your navel, and draw the eyes of your chest deep into their sockets. With an exhalation, lengthen the back of your arms toward your elbows, and lift up from the back edge of your respiratory diaphragm to come into the pose. (If you have difficulty straightening your arms, place your hands on blocks or on a wedge at the base of a wall. Use a strap around your elbows to keep your upper arms parallel.)

In Urdhva Dhanurasana, lengthen from the sides of your navel to your inner knees; simultaneously, lift your xiphoid process away from the back edge of your respiratory diaphragm. Broaden your midsternum so that it comes closer to the surface of your body and frees your midthoracic spine. At the same time, turn your manubrium toward the floor, and let it rest back into your body. Then draw the eyes of your chest

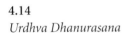

4.14
Urdhva Dhanurasana

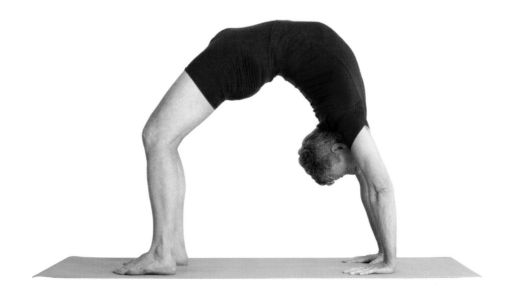

deep into their sockets, and lift your C7 away from your manubrium, to raise your head and release your cervical spine.

Maintain this position for another 30 seconds. Lift from your xiphoid process, broaden your midsternum, and turn your manubrium toward the floor. To come out of the pose, bend your knees, lower your pelvis to the floor, and rest with your knees bent. Repeat this pose three to six times.

RELATED POSE. Viparita Dandasana

MARICHYASANA III
POSE OF SAGE MARICHI III

PROPS

- 1 nonskid mat
- 1 blanket

This variation of Marichyasana III (Figure 4.15) helps to deepen the twist of the rib cage and shoulder girdle by balancing and turning from the sternum.

Fold a standard folded blanket in half or in thirds and place it lengthwise on your mat. Then sit at the front edge of the blanket with your legs extended. Bend your right knee and place your right foot on the floor directly in front of your right sitting bone. Lean back onto your right hand, and, with an inhalation, lengthen the sides of your navel away from your inner groins. With an exhalation, swing your left arm over your right knee, and turn your midsternum away from your right thigh to come into the pose. (If your left armpit comes in contact with your right thigh, you can wrap your left arm around your right leg, and take hold of your right wrist behind your back.)

4.15
Marichyasana III

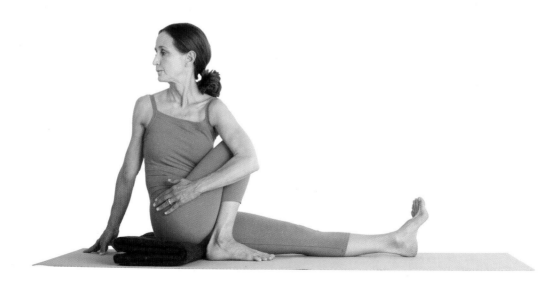

In Marichyasana III, lengthen down through your inner left leg, and lift the sides of your navel away from your inner groins. Then lift your xiphoid process away from the sides of your navel as you turn and broaden your midsternum to deepen the twist of your rib cage. Turn your manubrium away from your midsternum, and draw the eyes of your chest back into your body to release your shoulder girdle. Turn your head and neck to follow the movement of your right shoulder. Maintain this position for another 30 seconds, broadening your midsternum; then repeat to the other side.

RELATED POSES. Other sitting twists

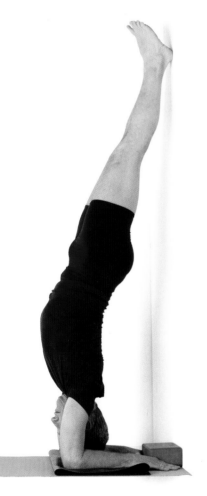

4.16a
*Pincha Mayurasana
at the Wall, Phase 1*

PINCHA MAYURASANA AT THE WALL
ELBOW BALANCE

PROPS
- 1 nonskid mat
- 1 block
- 1 wall

This variation of Pincha Mayurasana at the Wall has two phases. In the first, or beginner's, phase, your head hangs down and your spine is in a neutral position (Figure 4.16a). In the second, or final, phase, your head is lifted and your upper spine is arched, as in a backbend (Figure 4.16b).

Fold a nonskid mat in half or in thirds to provide a cushion for your forearms, and place the mat at the base of a wall. Kneeling in front of the mat, place your forearms on the mat with your palms facing down and your fingers pointing toward the wall. Use a block between your hands to prevent them from sliding together. Lengthen your index fingers against the sides of the block, and press your thumbs against the front of the block. Check that your forearms are parallel and that your elbows are directly below your shoulder joints. Then turn your toes under, lift your shins away from the floor, and straighten your legs.

As you walk your feet in toward your head, turn your xiphoid process toward the sides of your navel, and lengthen the back of your arms away from the eyes of your chest to stabilize your rib cage. With an inhalation, bring one leg in toward your chest with your knee bent. With an exhalation, swing the other leg up, keeping it perfectly straight. Let your bent leg be drawn up by the momentum of your straight leg; then rest both your heels on the wall with your legs extended.

Phase 1. In Pincha Mayurasana at the Wall, widen your collarbones and let your head hang freely between your upper arms. Lengthen the back of your arms away from the eyes of your chest, and lift the sides of your rib cage away from your inner elbows. Broaden your midsternum so that it faces directly forward. Then turn your xiphoid process toward the sides of your navel, and lift the center of your perineum away from the sides of your navel. Repeat these adjustments two or three times to create space in your shoulder joints and lengthen the sides of your chest.

Phase 2. To move into the second phase of Pincha Mayurasana at the Wall, lift the sides of your rib cage away from your inner elbows, and draw the eyes of your chest deep into their sockets. Then lift the crown of your head toward the wall, and turn your manubrium to face the floor. (If you have a shoulder imbalance, check that your manubrium is facing directly forward, and lift evenly from your outer collarbones.) Lift your manubrium into your body, turn your xiphoid process toward the sides of your navel, and lift the center of your perineum away from the sides of your navel. In making these adjustments, you may find that your legs are drawn away from the wall into a balancing position. If so, enjoy the achievement.

4.16b
*Pincha Mayurasana
at the Wall, Phase 2*

Remain in the pose for a few more breaths; then lengthen the back of your arms away from the eyes of your chest, turn your xiphoid process toward your navel, and draw your groins into your body as you lower your legs to the floor. Rest for a while in Adho Mukha Virasana (Child's Pose, Figure 3.11b).

Practice Notes. In Pincha Mayurasana at the Wall, start with your head down to open your shoulders and lift your xiphoid process. When your shoulders are open, lift your head and turn your manubrium toward the floor to facilitate balance. In the final pose, your manubrium and xiphoid process are turning away from each other, and your midsternum is broadening.

RELATED POSE. Adho Mukha Vrksasana

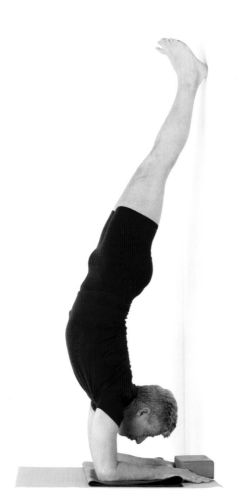

SALAMBA SIRSASANA
HEADSTAND

PROPS
• set up as determined in Chapter 2

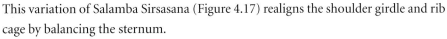

4.17
Salamba Sirsasana

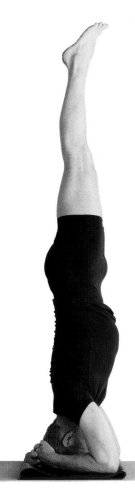

This variation of Salamba Sirsasana (Figure 4.17) realigns the shoulder girdle and rib cage by balancing the sternum.

Prepare for Salamba Sirsasana as described in Chapter 2. As you walk your feet in toward your head, press your xiphoid process into your rib cage, and lengthen the back of your arms away from the eyes of your chest. This action stabilizes your upper body, and prevents your weight from collapsing onto your neck as you raise your legs.

In Salamba Sirsasana, check the alignment of your sternum. If you have a shoulder imbalance or scoliosis, your manubrium may be turned slightly to the right or left. Adjust your manubrium so that it faces directly forward, and lift the sides of your rib cage away from your outer collarbones. Then stabilize your manubrium and adjust your midsternum so that it faces directly forward. Finally, bring the sides of your xiphoid process in line with the sides of your navel and lengthen your legs.

Maintain this position for 3 to 5 minutes. Soften the eyes of your chest, and draw them deep into their sockets as you lengthen the back of your arms toward your elbows. Let your manubrium release back into your body. At the same time, broaden your midsternum, so that your heart rests evenly between your spine and your lungs, neither pressing back onto the spine nor forward onto the lungs. If your lower ribs tend to protrude, turn your xiphoid process toward the sides of your navel, and lift your legs away from the sides of your respiratory diaphragm.

To come out of the pose, press your lower sternum into your rib cage, and lengthen the back of your arms away from the eyes of your chest, as you release your groins and bring your legs to the floor. Rest in Adho Mukha Virasana (Child's Pose, Figure 3.11b) for several breaths before continuing your practice.

RELATED POSES. Salamba Sirsasana variations

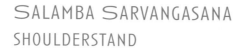

SALAMBA SARVANGASANA
SHOULDERSTAND

PROPS
• set up as determined in Chapter 1

Proper alignment of the sternum in Salamba Sarvangasana (Figure 4.18) helps to release your cervical spine and protect your neck.

Come into Salamba Sarvangasana as described in Chapter 1.

In Salamba Sarvangasana, relax your collarbones, widen your shoulders, and lengthen the back of your arms toward your elbows. Then broaden your midsternum, soften the eyes of your chest, and let your manubrium turn gently toward the floor. As the eyes of your chest sink deeper into their sockets, the back of your rib cage will naturally lift toward your waist. Take this opportunity to bring your hands higher on your upper back, and lift your legs away from your xiphoid process.

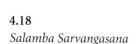

4.18
Salamba Sarvangasana

Remain in Salamba Sarvangasana for 3 to 10 minutes, or for as long as you can maintain the lift of the pose. Relax your upper thoracic spine, and lift from the sides of your chest. With the help of your arms, broaden your midsternum and draw the eyes of your chest deeper into their sockets. Then release your manubrium away from the base of your skull, so that your neck lengthens and your chin comes to meet your chest. Enjoy the pose. When you are ready, move into Halasana (Figure 4.19).

Practice Notes. When you press your manubrium toward your chin in Salamba Sarvangasana, your thoracic spine hardens, you feel tension at the base of your throat, and your neck is strained. In a well-balanced Salamba Sarvangasana, your midsternum moves forward, your manubrium turns toward the base of your throat and rests back into your body, and your chin comes to meet your chest.

RELATED POSES. Salamba Sarvangasana variations

HALASANA
PLOUGH POSE

PROPS
- set up as determined in Chapter 1

In this variation of Halasana (Figure 4.19), the xiphoid process turns toward the sides of the navel to release the lumbar spine.

To come into Halasana from Salamba Sarvangasana (Figure 4.18), press your xiphoid process into your rib cage, release your inner groins, and lower your legs to the floor. (If you have tight hamstrings or experience discomfort in your lower back, use a bolster, chair, or bench to support your feet.)

In Halasana, place your hands on the back of your rib cage with your palms flat. Draw the eyes of your chest deeper into your body, and lengthen the back of your arms toward your elbows. Turn your manubrium toward the floor, and broaden your midsternum, so that it comes gently forward. Turn your xiphoid process toward the sides of your navel, and lift the center of your perineum away from your navel. Release the base of your skull, relax your eyes, and soften the skin of your face.

Remain in Halasana for one-third to one-half the amount of time you spent in Salamba Sarvangasana. Then roll out of the pose; slide a few inches off your blankets, toward your head; and rest with your shoulders on the floor.

4.19
Halasana

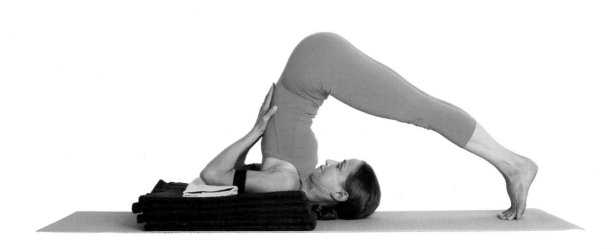

GARUDASANA FOR ARMS ONLY
EAGLE POSE VARIATION

PROPS
- 1 nonskid mat
- 1 blanket

This variation of Garudasana for Arms Only (Figure 4.20) releases your shoulders and upper back after Salamba Sarvangasana (Figure 4.18), and helps to balance your manubrium and midsternum.

Sit on your heels on a folded blanket with your knees together. (If you have knee problems, place a folded blanket between your calves and thighs or sit on a chair.) Raise your arms to shoulder level in front of you, with your palms facing each other. Cross your left arm over your right arm just above the elbow joint; then bend your elbows and entwine your forearms. Press your hands against each other by broadening your palms and lengthening your fingers, and raise your elbows to shoulder level with your forearms vertical. Let your chin descend to your sternal notch, and relax the base of your skull.

In Garudasana for Arms Only, check the alignment of your upper sternum and midsternum. First, turn your manubrium to face directly forward. Then, maintaining the position of your manubrium, turn your midsternum into the frontal plane. Feel how this adjustment alters the shape of your back rib cage. Finally, turn your xiphoid

4.20
*Garudasana
for Arms Only*

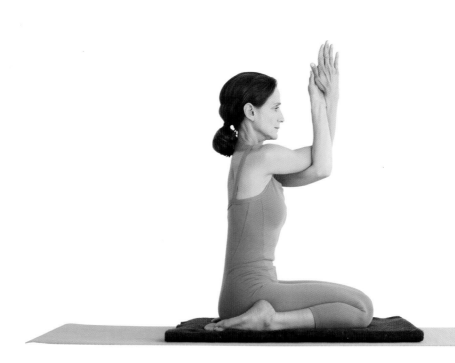

process toward the sides of your navel to broaden the back edge of your respiratory diaphragm, and deepen the stretch of your back rib cage. Maintain this position for several cycles of breath; then repeat to the other side.

Practice Notes. In Garudasana for Arms Only, the asymmetrical cross of your arms turns your manubrium and shoulder girdle away from the plane of your midsternum. The variation described here realigns your manubrium with your midsternum and minimizes the displacement of your shoulder girdle. Students with scoliosis should find this helpful, but will need to adapt these instructions to accommodate the difference between their two sides.

JANU SIRSASANA WITH HANDS ON BLOCKS
HEAD-OF-THE-KNEE POSE

PROPS
- 1 nonskid mat
- 2 blocks
- 1 blanket or wedge

OPTIONAL PROP
- 1 block or blanket

This variation of Janu Sirsasana with Hands on Blocks has two phases: a backbend phase, to lengthen the spine (Figure 4.21a), followed by a forward bend phase, to release the spine (Figure 4.21b).

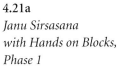

4.21a
*Janu Sirsasana
with Hands on Blocks,
Phase 1*

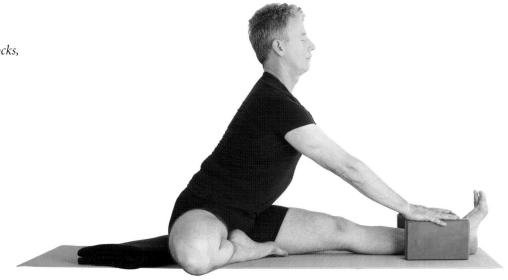

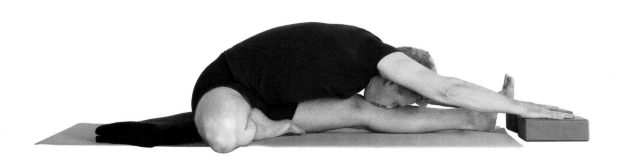

4.21b
*Janu Sirsasana
with Hands on Blocks,
Phase 2*

Place a folded blanket or wedge on your nonskid mat. Then sit with your sitting bones on the edge of the blanket or wedge and your legs extended. Bend your right leg and bring your right heel near your right groin with your knee out to the side. (If your right knee does not contact the floor, use a block or blanket to support the knee.)

Phase 1. Place a block on either side of your left foot. (If you are flexible, lay the blocks flat. If you have tight hamstrings, stand the blocks on end.) Then press your fingertips on the floor by your outer hips with your elbows bent. Draw your left groin back into your body, and turn your midsternum to face your left leg. With an inhalation, lift your xiphoid process away from the sides of your navel and raise your arms overhead. With an exhalation, keep your midsternum broad as you extend your torso over your left leg. Place your hands on blocks by the sides of your feet.

Maintain this position for several breaths. With each inhalation, broaden your midsternum; lift your xiphoid process away from the sides of your navel; and turn your manubrium toward your head, and let it rest back into your body. With each exhalation, maintain the length of your spine.

Phase 2. To move into the forward bend phase of Janu Sirsasana with Hands on Blocks, first, inhale and lift your xiphoid process away from the sides of your navel to lengthen your lumbar spine. Then, with an exhalation, turn your xiphoid process toward the sides of your navel, and let your chin drop toward your manubrium. At the same time, lengthen your arms away from the sides of your chest, and slide your blocks forward, if necessary, so that your arms remain fully extended.

Once you are deeper in your forward bend, turn your xyphoid process toward your left groin, and broaden your midsternum so that it comes directly over your left leg. Then soften the eyes of your chest, and extend your arms to lengthen the back of your body. Make sure that the eyes of your chest are equidistant from the floor, so that your shoulders are level. Drop your chin toward your sternal notch, and let your manubrium rest back into your body to release the base of your skull. Remain quietly in the pose for 1 to 2 minutes; then repeat to the other side.

Practice Notes. In the backbend phase of Janu Sirsasana with Hands on Blocks, your xiphoid process lifts away from the sides of your navel. In the forward bend phase, your xiphoid process turns toward the sides of your navel.

RELATED POSES. Paschimottanasana and other sitting forward bends

UJJAYI PRANAYAMA LYING
BASIC YOGA BREATHING

PROPS

- 1 nonskid mat
- 2 blankets

For this variation of Ujjayi Pranayama Lying (Figure 4.22), you need two blankets, placed one on top of the other to form a T shape. Fold the first blanket in half lengthwise to support your rib cage, and the second blanket in half crosswise to support your head and neck.

Lie on your back with your rib cage and waist supported by the first blanket. Adjust the second blanket so that it supports your head and neck comfortably, with your chin slightly tucked. (If you need more height under your head, fold your second blanket in thirds.) Extend your arms and legs as for Savasana (Figure 4.24) and close your eyes. Relax the skin of your face, move the back of your palate toward the crown of your head, and release any tightness at the base of your skull. Rest in this position for 2 to 3 minutes before you begin your breathing practice.

When you are ready, start with a deep, soft exhalation, observing the movement of your sternum and the flow of your breath. With an inhalation, broaden your midsternum and lift your xiphoid process away from the sides of your navel. Feel the area around your xiphoid process expanding evenly in all directions like the rays of the sun. At the same time, soften the eyes of your chest, so that your shoulders remain relaxed and the breath can move into your upper lungs.

With an exhalation, keep your midsternum broad and lengthen the sides of your navel down toward your inner groins as your xiphoid process slowly descends. Keep the eyes of your chest soft and broad, so that your shoulders do not tense. Repeat this cycle for 3 to 5 minutes, allowing your breath to build slowly and rhythmically with each inhalation. Then let your breath return to normal, and rest in Savasana for 1 to 2 minutes.

4.22
Ujjayi Pranayama Lying

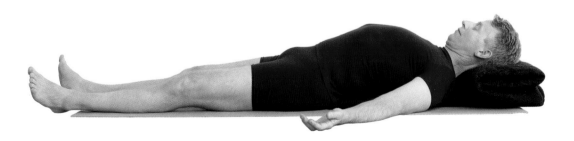

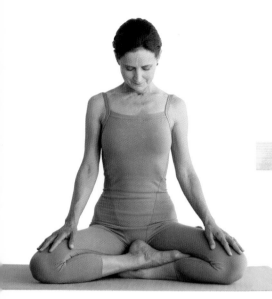

4.23
Siddhasana

UJJAYI PRANAYAMA SITTING
BASIC YOGA BREATHING

PROPS
- 1 nonskid mat
- 1 blanket

OPTIONAL PROPS
- 1 or 2 blocks or blankets
- 1 wedge

This variation of Ujjayi Pranayama Sitting focuses on the alignment and movement of the sternum.

Sit at the edge of a folded blanket in your most comfortable sitting position: Padmasana (Lotus Pose, Figure 3.21), Siddhasana (Perfect Pose, Figure 4.23), Sukhasana (Easy Pose, Figure 6.22), or Virasana (Hero Pose, Figure 5.24). If your knees are not in contact with the floor, use blocks or blankets to support them. (You can also use a wedge under your sitting bones to give an additional lift to your pelvis and spine.) Bring your elbows to the sides of your waist, and place your hands on your thighs with your palms turned down. Close your eyes gently and drop your chin to your sternal notch. Broaden your shoulders and release the base of your neck without collapsing your spine.

Begin with a deep, soft exhalation. With each inhalation, broaden the back edge of your respiratory diaphragm, and lift the sides of your rib cage. Expand the area around your xiphoid process evenly in all directions, as you broaden your midsternum and lift your xiphoid process away from the sides of your navel. At the same time, draw the eyes of your chest deeper into their sockets, and let your manubrium turn toward your head and rest back into your body. With each exhalation, keep your midsternum broad and lengthen the sides of your navel down toward your inner groins in time with your outgoing breath. Continue this cycle for 3 to 5 minutes; then change the cross of your legs, and repeat for another 3 to 5 minutes. When you are finished, rest in Savasana (Figure 4.24).

SAVASANA
RELAXATION POSE

PROP
- 1 nonskid mat

OPTIONAL PROP
- 1 blanket

This variation of Savasana (Figure 4.24) helps to keep your mind clear and alert by focusing on the sternum during inhalation and exhalation.

Lie on your back on a nonskid mat, with your knees bent and your feet on the floor in line with your sitting bones. (If the base of your skull feels tight, place a folded blanket under your head and neck.) Bend your elbows and press the back of your upper arms into the floor. Keep equal weight on your inner and outer elbows as you straighten your arms and rest the back of your hands on the floor. Then press your sacrum into the floor, and extend your legs, one at a time. Relax your pelvis and knees, and allow your legs to roll out.

Close your eyes and soften your inward gaze. With each inhalation, let your mid-sternum broaden. With each exhalation, let your xiphoid process slowly descend. With each cycle of breath, keep your mind alert, but allow your body to rest. Continue for 5 to 10 minutes.

When your body feels rested and your mind feels clear, bend your knees and turn onto your side before sitting up.

4.24
Savasana

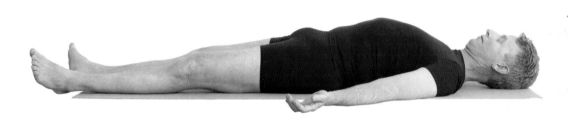

▶
PRACTICE SEQUENCE

TADASANA

TADASANA WITH A PARTNER

ADHO MUKHA SVANASANA

VIRABHADRASANA II

PADANGUSTHASANA

VIRABHADRASANA I

UTTANASANA

PARIVRTTA TIKONASANA

URDHVA MUKHA SVANASANA

USTRASANA

URDHVA DHANURASANA

MARICHYASANA III

PINCHA MAYURASANA AT THE WALL

SALAMBA SIRSASANA

SALAMBA SARVANGASANA

HALASANA

GARUDASANA FOR ARMS ONLY

JANU SIRSASANA WITH HANDS ON BLOCKS

UJJAY PRANAYAMA LYING

UJJAY PRANAYAMA SITTING

SAVASANA

5 COLLARBONES, KIDNEYS, AND GROINS

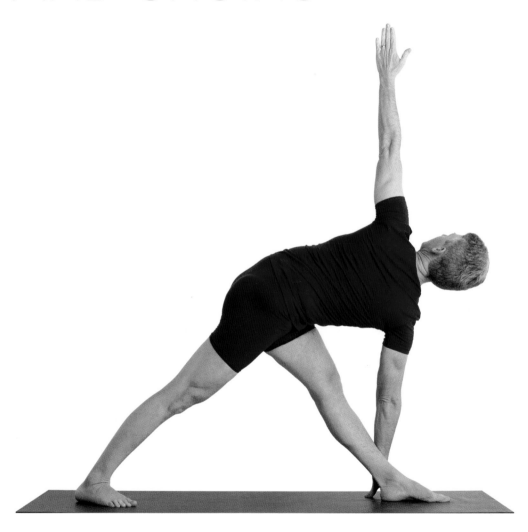

IN THIS CHAPTER, we explore the subtle relationship between the inner groins, the kidneys, and the collarbones. By integrating the movement of the inner groins (at the front edge of the pelvic diaphragm) with the movement of the kidneys (at the back edge of the respiratory diaphragm) and with the movement of the collarbones (at the front edge of the thoracic diaphragm), we bring freedom and vitality to the whole of the upper body.

▶
INNER GROINS

Anatomically, the groin is the groove, or crease, between the lower abdomen and the upper thigh that follows the line of the front hip joint. The groin area is protected by the inguinal ligament, which runs from the crest of the pelvis (anterior superior iliac spine) to the pubic bone. The groin area is composed of outer groins and inner groins—the outer groins being farther away from, and the inner groins closer to, the pubic bone.

In yoga, the inner groins have a special significance because of their relation to the deeper muscles of the body. When I speak of the "inner groins," I refer in particular to the circular hollows, or indentations, you can feel with your fingertips at the very tops of your inner thighs—between the sides of the pubic bone and the upper thighbones. The muscles and ligaments surrounding and underlying these indentations I call the inner groin muscles, or, more simply, the inner groins. The major muscles that pass through this area are the psoas and iliacus (Figure 5.1).

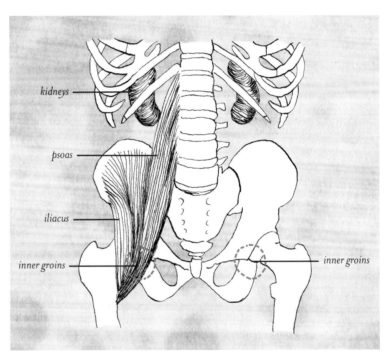

5.1
*The Psoas
and Iliacus Muscles*

The psoas and iliacus are the deep abdominal muscles that help to stabilize the spine and the pelvis internally. The psoas originates from the dome of the respiratory diaphragm and from all vertebrae from T12 to L5, travels through the pelvic basin, and passes over the pubic bone before inserting on the lesser trochanter of the thighbone. The iliacus originates from the interior walls at the sides of the pelvis and from the ligaments of the lumbar-sacral joint and the sacroiliac joints. A portion of the iliacus inserts on the tendon of the psoas, and the rest crosses over the pubic bone and inserts on the lesser trochanter. The psoas and iliacus are so closely allied in form and function that they are often referred to as the iliopsoas.

Any movement of the inner groins directly affects the quality and movement of the psoas and iliacus and the position of the pelvis. In poses where you want to lift your pelvis away from your thighs, such as Tadasana (Figure 5.5), you should broaden and lengthen your inner groins in order to firm and stabilize your iliopsoas. In poses where you want to bring your pelvis toward your thighs, such as Uttanasana (Figure 5.10), you need to relax your inner groins and draw them deeper into your body in order to release your iliopsoas.

If you are unfamiliar with the movement of the inner groins, try this exercise. Stand in Tadasana with your feet a few inches apart. Press your fingertips into the hollows on either side of your pubic bone. With an inhalation, lift your pelvis away from your inner thighs, and feel the groin muscles underneath your fingertips firm and lengthen. With an exhalation, relax your inner groins and draw them back, up, and over your fingertips to release your pelvis into a forward bend. (For a further discussion of the movement of the inner groins, see "Practice Notes" for Adho Mukha Svanasana as described for Figure 5.6.)

In asymmetrical poses, such as Utthita Parsvakonasana (Figure 3.5), your right and left inner groins function differently because one side of your body is bending forward as in Uttanasana, and the other side is extended, as in Tadasana. In Utthita Parsvakonasana to the right, for example, let your right inner groin release and draw deeper into your body to bring your pelvis toward the thigh of your bent leg. At the same time, broaden and lengthen through your inner left groin to lift your pelvis away from your extended leg.

▶
KIDNEYS

The kidneys are a filtering system that purifies the blood by removing waste and excess fluid, thereby restoring vital energy. Protected by the floating ribs at the back of the body, the kidneys are positioned near the sides of the spine at the critical thoracolumbar junction. The right kidney is slightly lower than the left kidney. The upper halves of the kidneys are parallel with the lower thoracic vertebrae (T11–T12) and the lower halves of the kidneys with the upper lumbar vertebrae (L1–L2). The kidneys lie in close proximity to the psoas, with the kidneys posterior to, or behind, the spine and the psoas anterior to, or in front, of the spine. With each cycle of breath, the kidneys slide up and down the track of the psoas, as if on rails (Figure 5.2).

The proximity of the kidneys to the psoas explains the vital connection between the inner groins and the kidneys. When you lift your kidneys away from your inner groins, as in Tadasana, you are, in effect, lengthening your psoas by stabilizing the lower end at the inner groins, and lifting the upper end through focus on the kidneys. For inverted poses, such as Adho Mukha Svanasana (Figure 5.6), the instruction is

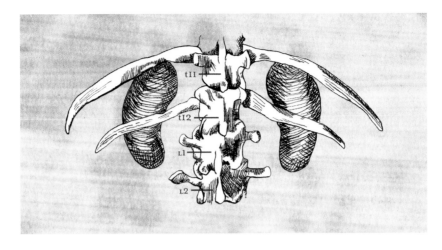

5.3
*Alignment of the Kidneys
with the Back Body*

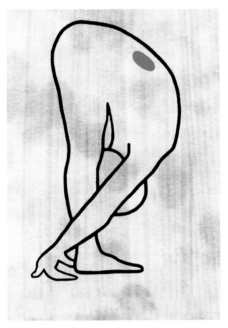

reversed: you lift your inner groins away from your kidneys to lengthen the psoas, because you are working against gravity.

The lift of your kidneys away from your inner groins is described as a linear movement, but, in reality, it is a three-dimensional one. When you lift your kidneys away from your inner groins in Tadasana, your kidneys not only lift up toward your thoracic spine, but the front of your kidneys also turn upward, so that your lower kidneys move deeper into your body, and your upper kidneys rest back against your rib cage. This is the optimal position for the kidneys when you want to extend the spine.

When you want to release the spine into a forward bend, as in Uttanasana, the direction of your kidneys is reversed. In forward bends, let the front of your kidneys turn down toward the lumbar spine, so that your upper kidneys move deeper into your body and your lower kidneys rest back against your floating ribs (Figure 5.3).

No matter what pose you are practicing, your kidneys should always turn in the same direction as your rib cage. If your rib cage turns up but your kidneys turn down, your backbends will be limited. If your rib cage turns down but your kidneys turn up, your forward bends will be restricted. In all poses, adjust your kidneys so that they lie parallel to the surface of your back rib cage. If the internal organs of your inner body are not properly aligned with the musculoskeletal system of your outer body, the movement of your spine will be compromised.

The kidneys move in all three dimensions: they lift up and down, turn forward and back, and move closer to or farther away from the spine. When your kidneys move closer to the spine, they also turn toward the spine. When your kidneys move away from the spine, they also turn away from the spine. This lateral movement of the kidneys is most evident in twisting poses. When you turn your rib cage to the right, lift your left kidney away from your left groin, but turn it toward your lumbar spine. At the same time, lengthen your right kidney away from your right groin, and turn it away from your thoracic spine. Both kidneys turn and both kidneys lengthen, but your left kidney turns more, and your right kidney lengthens more. (Reverse these directions when turning your rib cage to the left.)

A word of caution: try not to initiate the turn of your kidneys by gripping your diaphragm. Let the front edge of your diaphragm remain soft and broad, so that the movement of your kidneys comes from the core of your body, not from the surface. To encourage this internal movement, visualize the shape and position of your kidneys in relation to your spine and rib cage. Be aware of the quality of energy in your kidneys. If your kidneys feel as hard and dry as walnuts, your energy is *rajasic* (overactive). If they feel as heavy as overripe melons, your energy is *tamasic* (lethargic.) When your kidneys feel as firm and juicy as ripe mangoes, your energy is *sattvic* (balanced and replenishing).

▶
COLLARBONES

The collarbones, or clavicles, are long, slender, gently curving bones that rest on the upper front rib cage and form part of the shoulder girdle. The inner corner of the collarbone is attached to the manubrium, or upper sternum, via the sterno-clavicular joint. The space, or indentation, between the inner collarbones is called the sternal

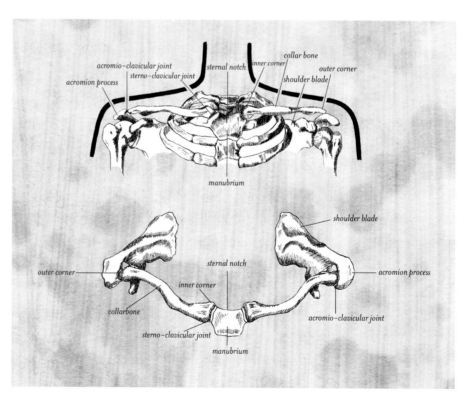

5.4
Collarbones

notch. The outer corner of the collarbone is attached to the acromion process of the scapula, or shoulder blade, via the acromio-clavicular joint. The acromion process is the bony protruberance you feel when you run your fingertips along the ridge of your outer shoulder (Figure 5.4).

The collarbones are especially vulnerable to accident and injury. Apart from the feet, no other bones of the body are broken so frequently. A fall from your bicycle, a skiing mishap, or any heavy impact to your shoulder can force the collarbone out of alignment. Most often, the collarbone is pushed into the body, stressing the sterno-clavicular joint and constricting the shoulder. In fact, many shoulder problems can be diminished or resolved by realigning and balancing the collarbones.

In Tadasana, widen your collarbones away from your sternal notch and broaden your shoulders evenly. In inverted poses, such as Adho Mukha Svanasana (Figure 5.6) and Salamba Sirsasana (Figure 5.16), check that your right collarbone moves to the right and your left collarbone to the left, so that your weight is distributed evenly on your arms. In Salamba Sarvangasana (Figure 5.18), remember to release your collarbones away from your sternal notch, rather than pull them with the force of your arms.

In addition to the lateral movement of your collarbones, there is also a circular movement. When you raise your arms overhead, your collarbones roll up toward your head to initiate the movement. On the other hand, when you extend your arms behind your back, your collarbones naturally roll down, or away from your head. Rolling your collarbones up takes your spine into a backbend, and draws your head and shoulders back. Rolling your collarbones down releases your spine into a forward bend, and brings your head and shoulders forward.

In asymmetrical poses, you will find that one collarbone needs to roll up, while the other one rolls down. For example, when twisting to the right in Marichyasana III (Figure 4.15), first, let your collarbones release away from your sternal notch, as in Tadasana. Then roll your right collarbone up, to draw your right shoulder back, and roll your left collarbone down, to bring your left shoulder forward. (The right side of your body moves into a backbend and the left side into a forward bend.)

When rolling your collarbones up toward your head, broaden your midsternum to lift your upper ribs; roll your sternal notch toward the base of your throat; and lengthen your collarbones from the inner corners to the outer corners. When your arms are raised overhead, as in Urdhva Hastasana I (Figure 7.6), your collarbones should form a long, narrow V pressing in toward the median line of your body and lifting up through your inner arms.

When rolling your collarbones down, or away from your head, roll down from the outer corner of the collarbone. Before rolling your outer collarbone down, take a moment to relax the acromio-clavicular joint, where your outer collarbone meets the acromion process of your shoulder blade. When the acromio-clavicular joint is locked, the movement of your shoulder joint may be seriously impeded, especially in Adho Mukha Svanasana and other inverted poses. Create space in your acromio-clavicular joints to free your shoulders.

When rolling your inner collarbones up, do not pull your outer collarbones back.

This action squeezes your shoulder blades into your spine and narrows the back of your rib cage. When rolling your outer collarbones down, do not push your outer collarbones forward. This action pulls your shoulder blades away from your back rib cage and narrows your front rib cage.

The following practice sequence integrates the movement of your collarbones, kidneys, and groins. Placing these three areas of the body in dialogue with one another helps to align and nourish your poses at the deepest level.

5.5
Tadasana

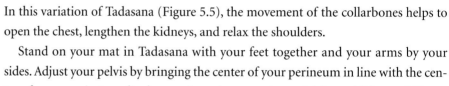

TADASANA
MOUNTAIN POSE

PROP
• 1 nonskid mat

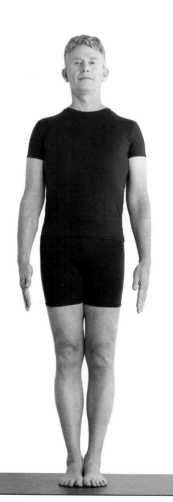

In this variation of Tadasana (Figure 5.5), the movement of the collarbones helps to open the chest, lengthen the kidneys, and relax the shoulders.

Stand on your mat in Tadasana with your feet together and your arms by your sides. Adjust your pelvis by bringing the center of your perineum in line with the center of your respiratory diaphragm. Lengthen your inner thighs and lift your kidneys away from your inner groins. Keep the back edge of your respiratory diaphragm broad, but let your kidneys move closer to the spine. If one kidney drops away from the spine, adjust your pose so that both kidneys lift evenly.

Then relax your shoulders, broaden your midsternum, and widen your collarbones away from your sternal notch. Move your outer collarbones toward your inner arms, and let your inner collarbones roll gently up toward your head.

Remain in Tadasana for another 30 seconds. Lengthen your inner thighs, lift your kidneys away from your inner groins, and widen your collarbones away from the sternal notch. Feel how these adjustments support and enhance one another. Return to Tadasana after each standing pose.

Practice Notes. Remember to release your collarbones away from your sternal notch in a lateral direction, so that the top edges of your shoulder blades can widen as well. When you pull your outer collarbones toward the back of your body, you squeeze your shoulder blades toward your spine and narrow your upper back. Let the front and back of your rib cage be equally broad!

ADHO MUKHA SVANASANA
DOWNWARD-FACING DOG POSE

PROP

- 1 nonskid mat

In this variation of Adho Mukha Svanasana (Figure 5.6), roll your collarbones away from your head to open your shoulders and lengthen your spine.

Begin on your mat in Adho Mukha Virasana with Arms Extended (Child's Pose Variation, Figure 3.4b), with your pelvis resting on your heels and your arms extended forward. Place your hands on the mat with the mounds of your thumbs in line with the center of your shoulder joints, so that your upper arms are parallel to each other. In this position, draw your groins into your body, lengthen from your kidneys toward your arms, and roll the outer corners of your collarbones away from your head. Feel the stretch at the back of your body! Then come up onto your hands and knees, without changing the position of your hands. Turn your toes under, lengthen the back of your kidneys, and lift your groins into your body as you raise your pelvis and straighten your legs.

In Adho Mukha Svanasana, relax the outer corners of your collarbones to create space in your acromio-clavicular joints. Check that the outer corners of your collarbones are equidistant from the floor. If one side sinks lower than the other, adjust the outer corners of your collarbones, so that they are both directly in line with your inner arms. Then lengthen your collarbones away from your inner arms, so that they form a long, narrow V pointing toward your sternum. At the same time, turn the front of your kidneys toward your pelvis, and draw your inner groins into your body to lengthen your psoas.

5.6

Adho Mukha Svanasana

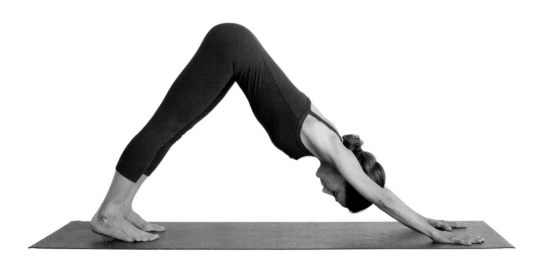

Remain in Adho Mukha Svanasana for 1 to 2 minutes. Continue to roll the outer corners of your collarbones gently away from your head, and lengthen through your inner arms. Lift your rib cage away from your shoulders by turning the front of your kidneys toward your pelvis and drawing your groins deep into your body. To come out of the pose, bend your knees and rest in Adho Mukha Virasana (Child's Pose, Figure 3.11b).

Practice Notes. In order to lengthen your kidneys in Adho Mukha Svanasana, you need to find just the right angle to lift your groins into your body. This angle lies somewhere between directly up and directly back, and depends upon your body type and flexibility. If you have tighter hip joints, you need to lift your groins more up than back. If you are overly flexible, you need to move your groins more back than up. When you find just the right angle between up and back for your particular body, your kidneys will feel energized and will lengthen easily.

In order to lengthen your kidneys in other poses, such as Padangusthasana (Figure 5.8), Uttanasana (Figure 5.10), Prasarita Padottanasana (Figure 2.13a), or Paschimottanasana (Figure 5.21), you will again need to find just the right angle to draw your groins into your body. Be aware that this angle may differ from pose to pose, and from day to day. You will know when you have found just the right angle by the energizing effect on your kidneys.

5.7
Utthita Trikonasana

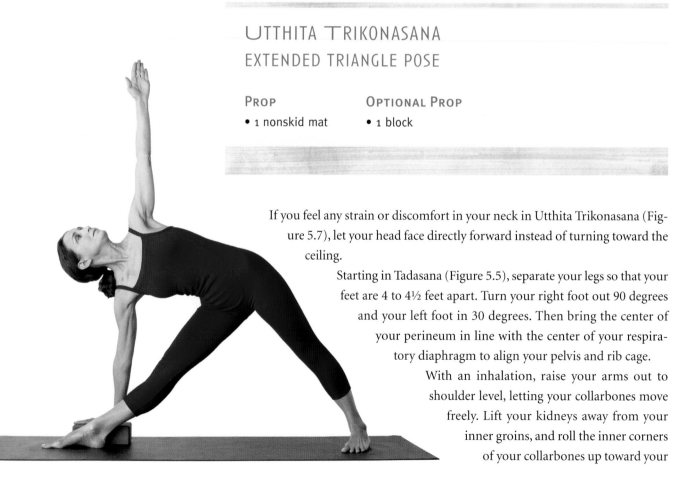

UTTHITA TRIKONASANA
EXTENDED TRIANGLE POSE

PROP
• 1 nonskid mat

OPTIONAL PROP
• 1 block

If you feel any strain or discomfort in your neck in Utthita Trikonasana (Figure 5.7), let your head face directly forward instead of turning toward the ceiling.

Starting in Tadasana (Figure 5.5), separate your legs so that your feet are 4 to 4½ feet apart. Turn your right foot out 90 degrees and your left foot in 30 degrees. Then bring the center of your perineum in line with the center of your respiratory diaphragm to align your pelvis and rib cage.

With an inhalation, raise your arms out to shoulder level, letting your collarbones move freely. Lift your kidneys away from your inner groins, and roll the inner corners of your collarbones up toward your head. With an exhalation, draw your right inner groin into your body as you extend your torso over your right leg. Place your right hand or fingertips on the floor by your outer right ankle. (Use a block under your hand if you can't reach the floor easily.)

In Utthita Trikonasana, lift your right kidney away from your right inner groin, and turn it toward your lumbar spine to give support. Lift your left kidney away from your left inner groin, and turn it away from your thoracic spine to open your chest. Release your collarbones away from your sternal notch. Roll the outer corner of your right collarbone down to bring your right shoulder forward; at the same time, lengthen from your right collarbone to your inner right arm. Roll the inner corner of your left collarbone up to bring your left shoulder back; at the same time, lengthen from your left collarbone to your inner left arm.

Hold Utthita Trikonasana for another 30 seconds. Lift your kidneys away from your inner groins, and broaden your collarbones away from your sternal notch so that your head hangs freely. To come out of the pose, lift your kidneys away from your groins. Repeat to the other side.

RELATED POSES. Ardha Chandrasana, Utthita Parsvakonasana

PADANGUSTHASANA
TOE-HOLDING POSE

5.8
Padangusthasana

PROP
• 1 nonskid mat

OPTIONAL PROP
• 1 block

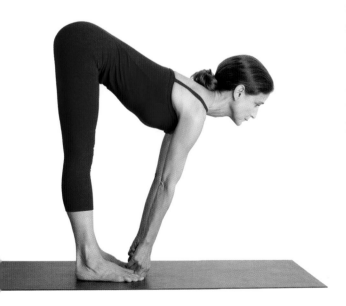

In this variation of Padangusthasana (Figure 5.8), roll the inner corners of your collarbones toward your head to release your thoracic spine and lengthen your kidneys, as in a backbend.

Stand on your mat in Tadasana (Figure 5.5) with your feet a few inches apart. Place your hands on your hips with your thumbs pressing down on your sacrum. Roll your inner collarbones toward your head, and let your head drop back. At the same time, broaden your outer collarbones toward your inner arms, and bring your upper arms parallel to each other. With an inhalation, lift your kidneys toward your thoracic spine. With an exhalation, draw your groins into your body to release your hip joints, and bring your torso parallel to the floor, maintaining the length of your kidneys. Then extend your arms and wrap your second and third fingers around your big toes. (If you cannot reach your toes without rounding your back, place a block on end directly in front of your feet to support your hands.)

In Padangusthasana, draw your groins into your body at just the right angle to release and lengthen your kidneys toward your thoracic spine. Widen your sternal notch and roll your inner collarbones up toward your head to release your thoracic spine. Then widen your outer collarbones toward your inner arms, and lift your head from the base of your skull.

Maintain this position for several breaths, integrating the movement of your collarbones, kidneys, and groins to maximize the length of your spine. To come out of the pose, place your hands on your hips, and, with an inhalation, lift your torso from the strength of your thoracic spine. With an exhalation, extend your arms by your sides and return to Tadasana.

RELATED POSE. Prasarita Padottanasana (Phase 1)

5.9
Virabhadrasana I

VIRABHADRASANA I
WARRIOR I POSE

PROP
• 1 nonskid mat

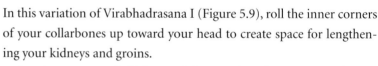

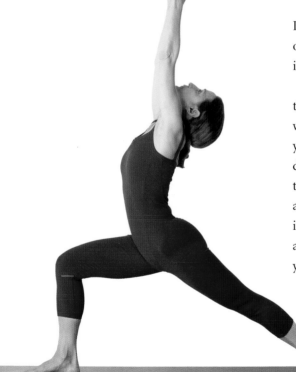

In this variation of Virabhadrasana I (Figure 5.9), roll the inner corners of your collarbones up toward your head to create space for lengthening your kidneys and groins.

Stand on your mat in Tadasana (Figure 5.5), and separate your legs so that your feet are about 3½ feet apart. Place your hands on your hips, with your thumbs pressing the top edge of your sacrum on either side of your spine. Turn your right foot out 90 degrees, and your left foot in 60 degrees. Then lift your kidneys away from your groins, and turn your torso to face your right leg. Draw your right groin back into your body, and roll your left groin in, so that your inner groins are parallel. With an inhalation, raise your arms overhead and lengthen through your inner arms. With an exhalation, move your left groin forward as you bend your right knee to form a right angle.

In Virabhadrasana I, lift your kidneys away from your inner groins. Lengthen your right kidney up toward your thoracic spine, and turn your left kidney toward your lumbar spine. Roll the inner corners of your collarbones away from your midsternum, and lift the outer corners of your collarbones as you lengthen your inner arms. Then turn your sternal notch toward the base of your throat and let your head drop back, but only if it feels comfortable on your neck. Soften your eyes, relax your jaw, and lift your C7 deeper into your body.

Maintain this position for 30 seconds. Lift your kidneys away from your inner groins, roll the inner corners of your collarbones up, and lengthen through your inner arms. To come out of the pose, lift from your kidneys and groins with an inhalation, and bring your arms down with an exhalation. Repeat to the other side.

UTTANASANA
STANDING FORWARD BEND

PROP
• 1 nonskid mat

OPTIONAL PROP
• 1 block

5.10
Uttanasana

In this variation of Uttanasana (Figure 5.10), roll the outer corners of your collarbones away from your head to deepen your forward bend.

Start in Tadasana (Figure 5.5) with your feet a few inches apart. With an inhalation, roll your collarbones up toward your head as you bring your arms forward and raise them overhead. Turn your palms to face each other, and lift the outer corners of your collarbones to lengthen through your inner arms. With an exhalation, draw your inner groins back into your body to release your hip joints and lengthen your kidneys toward your thoracic spine as you extend your torso forward. Place your hands on the floor by the sides of your feet, so that your upper arms are parallel to each other. (Use a block under your hands if you cannot reach the floor easily.)

In Uttanasana, draw your inner groins into your body at just the right angle to allow the back of your kidneys to lengthen toward your head. Turn the front of your kidneys toward your inner groins, so that your lower kidneys rest against your lower ribs and your upper kidneys move deeper into your body. Then widen your sternal notch to release your head and neck. Roll your collarbones away from your head to bring your shoulders forward, and lengthen from the outer corners of your collarbones to your inner elbows. Draw your eyes deep into their sockets, and relax the base of your skull.

Maintain this position for about 30 seconds. Continue to lift your groins, lengthen your kidneys, and release your collarbones away from the sternal notch. To come out of the pose, place your hands on your hips, and roll your collarbones up as you raise your head. With an inhalation, lift your torso from the strength of your thoracic spine. With an exhalation, lengthen your arms by the sides of your body and return to Tadasana.

RELATED POSE. Prasarita Padottanasana (Phase 2)

PARIVRTTA TRIKONASANA
REVOLVED TRIANGLE POSE

5.11
Parivrtta Trikonasana

PROP	**OPTIONAL PROP**
• 1 nonskid mat	• 1 block

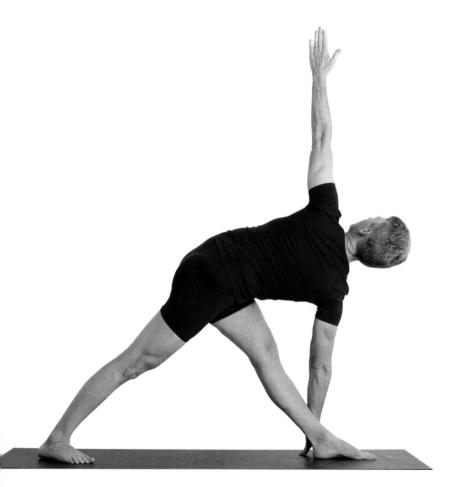

In Parivrtta Trikonasana (Figure 5.11), one kidney turns toward the spine, and the other kidney lengthens to deepen the twist.

Start in Tadasana (Figure 5.5), and separate your feet 4 feet apart. Place your hands on your hips, and turn your right foot out 90 degrees and your left foot in 60 degrees. Lift your kidneys away from your groins, and turn your pelvis to face your right leg. Then draw your right groin back into your body, and roll your left groin in, so that your inner groins are parallel to each other.

With an inhalation, raise your left arm overhead, and lift the outer corner of your left collarbone toward your inner left arm to stretch the left side of your rib cage. At the same time, turn your left kidney toward your spine, and lift it away from your left inner groin. With an exhalation, lengthen your right kidney away from your right groin, and extend your torso over your right leg. Place your left hand on the floor directly below your left shoulder, and extend your right arm toward the ceiling. (Use a block under your left hand, if necessary, so that your spine is parallel to the floor.)

In Parivrtta Trikonasana, lift your kidneys away from your inner groins, turning your left kidney toward your lumbar spine and lengthening your right kidney toward your thoracic spine. Then widen your sternal notch and relax your collarbones. Roll your left collarbone down to bring your left shoulder forward, and lengthen from the outer corner of your collarbone through your inner left arm. Roll your right collarbone up to bring your right shoulder back, and lengthen from the outer corner of your collarbone through your inner right arm.

Maintain this position for 30 seconds. Lengthen through your inner left groin to keep your left leg strong. Turn your left kidney toward your lumbar spine, and lengthen your right kidney toward your thoracic spine. Keep your collarbones soft and broad as you lengthen your inner arms. To come out of the pose, lift your torso away from your groins. Repeat to the other side.

RELATED POSE. Parivrtta Ardha Chandrasana

5.12
Pincha Mayurasana at the Wall

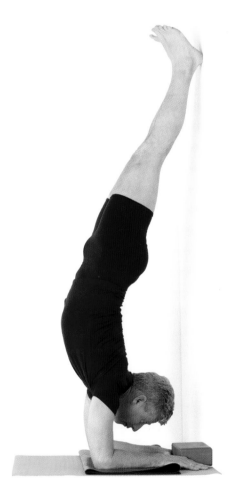

PINCHA MAYURASANA AT THE WALL
ELBOW BALANCE

PROPS

- 1 nonskid mat
- 1 block
- 1 wall

This variation of Pincha Mayurasana at the Wall (Figure 5.12) creates mobility in your thoracic spine by releasing your collarbones and lengthening your kidneys.

Place a nonskid mat folded in half or in quarters at the base of a wall. Put a block on the mat against the wall to separate and stabilize your hands. Then kneel in front of the mat, and position your hands so that your index fingers press the sides of the block, your thumbs press the front edge of the block, and your palms lie flat.

With an inhalation, broaden your collarbones and lengthen your kidneys. With an exhalation, lift your inner groins into your body as you raise your pelvis and straighten your legs. With another inhalation, bend one knee and step your foot closer to the wall so that your thigh almost touches your chest. With an exhalation, keep your other leg perfectly straight as you swing it in a wide arc toward the wall. Let the momentum of your straight leg draw your bent leg away from the floor. Rest your heels on the wall with your legs extended, and lift your inner groins away from your kidneys.

In Pincha Mayurasana at the Wall, roll the inner corners of your collarbones toward your head, deepen your sternal notch, and lift your head toward the wall without tightening the base of your skull. Move your outer collarbones toward your inner arms, and lift the sides of your rib cage away from your inner elbows. (If you have a shoulder imbalance, make sure that your outer collarbones are in line with the frontal plane of your body.) Then let your liver and stomach rest back onto your kidneys. Lift your kidneys away from your thoracic spine, and lift your inner groins away from your kidneys as you lengthen your legs. Do not be surprised if your legs come away from the wall!

Maintain this position for 30 seconds. To come out of the pose, lift your outer collarbones, lengthen your kidneys, and draw your inner groins into your body as you lower your legs. Rest for several breaths in Adho Mukha Virasana (Child's Pose, Figure 3.11b).

RELATED POSE. Adho Mukha Vrksasana

SALABHASANA
LOCUST POSE

PROPS
- 1 nonskid mat
- 1 blanket

5.13
Salabhasana

In Salabhasana (Figure 5.13), keep your arms parallel to the floor throughout the pose to protect your lower back.

Lie face down with a folded blanket under your pelvis and your forehead touching the floor. Extend your arms by the sides of your body, with your palms facing up. Then, raising your head, lift both your shoulders and your hands away from the floor so that your arms are parallel to the floor. To focus the work in your upper back, roll

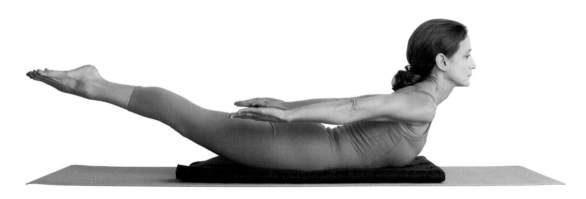

your inner collarbones up and draw your kidneys into your body, lifting your kidneys toward your thoracic spine. At the same time, lift your inner groins away from your kidneys to raise your legs and strengthen your lower abdomen.

In Salabhasana, release the inner corners of your collarbones away from the sternal notch and soften your kidneys. Widen the outer corners of your collarbones toward your inner arms, and lengthen your inner groins. Maintain this position for several breaths; then release with an exhalation. Repeat two or three times.

RELATED POSES. Ustrasana, Urdhva Mukha Svanasana, other backbends

URDHVA DHANURASANA
UPWARD-FACING BOW POSE

PROP
- 1 nonskid mat

OPTIONAL PROPS
- 1 strap
- 1 wedge
- 2 blocks

5.14
Urdhva Dhanurasana

In Urdhva Dhanurasana (Figure 5.14), move your kidneys away from your inner groins to lift your rib cage, and lengthen your inner groins away from your kidneys to raise your pelvis.

Lie on your back on a nonskid mat with your knees bent and your feet flat on the floor in line with your sitting bones. Raise your arms overhead and place your hands flat on the floor in line with your outer shoulders. With an inhalation, relax your

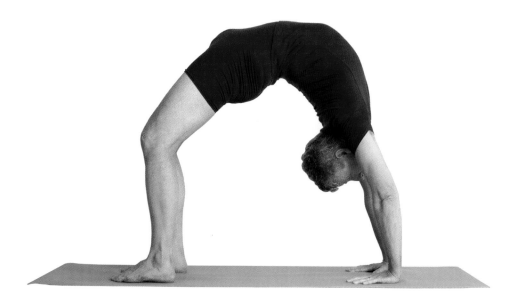

shoulders, roll the inner corners of your collarbones toward your head, and lengthen from the outer corners of your collarbones toward your inner elbows. With an exhalation, turn your kidneys away from your inner groins as you lift your rib cage and pelvis away from the floor. (If your arms do not straighten easily, use a strap around your elbows for support. If you experience discomfort in your wrists, use a wedge or blocks under your hands.)

In Urdhva Dhanurasana, roll the inner corners of your collarbones toward your head, and lengthen the sides of your rib cage. Turn your sternal notch toward the base of your throat, and lift your head from the base of your skull. Lift your kidneys away from your inner groins; at the same time, lengthen your liver and stomach toward your inner groins to prevent them from pressing against and constricting your lungs. If your pelvis drops lower than your rib cage, lengthen your inner groins away from your kidneys. If your rib cage drops lower than your pelvis, lift your kidneys away from your groins.

Maintain this position for 30 seconds. Roll the inner corners of your collarbones toward your head, turn the front of your kidneys away from your inner groins, and lengthen your inner groins away from your kidneys and toward your feet. If you have a shoulder imbalance, make sure that your outer collarbones are in line with the frontal plane of your body. To come out of the pose, bend your knees and press your shinbones forward. Rest with your back on the floor and your knees bent until your breath returns to normal. Repeat three to six times.

RELATED POSE. Viparita Dandasana

PARIVRTTA UTTANASANA
REVOLVED STANDING FORWARD BEND

PROP
• 1 nonskid mat

OPTIONAL PROP
• 1 block

Parivrtta Uttanasana (Figure 5.15) relieves tightness in the lower back, neutralizes the spine, and is a good counterpose after practicing backbends.

Come into Uttanasana as described for Figure 5.10. Extend your right arm forward, with your hand on the floor in line with your right shoulder. (Use a block under your right hand if your hamstrings are tight.) Bend your left arm and take hold of your outer right calf with your left hand so that your left forearm is parallel to the floor. Then relax your diaphragm and stabilize your inner groins. Turn your left kidney toward your lumbar spine, and lengthen your outer left collarbone toward your inner

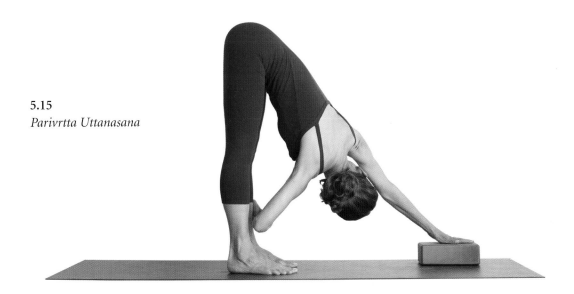

5.15
Parivrtta Uttanasana

5.16
Salamba Sirsasana

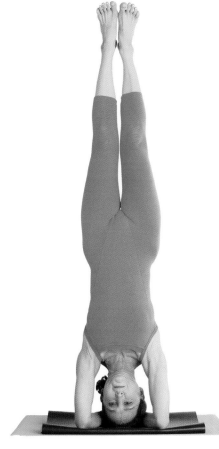

left arm. At the same time, lift your outer right collarbone toward your inner right arm, and turn your right kidney away from your thoracic spine.

Maintain this position for 30 seconds. Keep your inner groins level to stabilize your pelvis. Turn your left kidney toward your lumbar spine, and your right kidney away from your thoracic spine. Release your collarbones away from your sternal notch. Then return to Uttanasana, and repeat to the other side.

SALAMBA SIRSASANA
HEADSTAND

PROPS

• set up as determined in Chapter 2

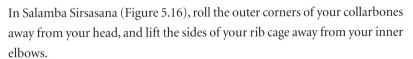

In Salamba Sirsasana (Figure 5.16), roll the outer corners of your collarbones away from your head, and lift the sides of your rib cage away from your inner elbows.

Prepare for Salamba Sirsasana as described in Chapter 2. Once you have placed your forearms and the crown of your head on your blanket, turn your toes under, draw your groins into your body, and straighten your legs. As you walk your feet closer to your head, roll the outer corners of your collarbones away from your head to protect your neck, and lift your inner groins away from your kidneys. Come up with either bent knees or straight legs, depending on your flexibility and strength.

In Salamba Sirsasana, release your collarbones away from your sternal notch. Move your right collarbone toward your right arm and your left collarbone toward your left arm, so that your weight is balanced evenly. Then press down on your elbows, move the outer corners of your collarbones toward your inner arms, and lift the sides of your rib cage. Let your liver and stomach rest back against your kidneys, and lift your kidneys away from your thoracic spine. Then lift your inner groins away from your kidneys and lengthen your legs. Let the weight of your legs balance evenly between your inner groins, at the front of your body, and your kidneys, at the back of your body.

Maintain this position for 3 to 5 minutes. Check that the outer corners of your collarbones are in line with the frontal plane of your body. Then roll the outer corners of your collarbones away from your head, and lift the sides of your rib cage away from your inner elbows. To come out of the pose, draw your groins into your body, lengthen your kidneys, and lift your outer collarbones away from your head as you lower your legs. Rest for several breaths in Adho Mukha Virasana (Child's Pose, Figure 3.11b).

RELATED POSES. Salamba Sirsasana variations

SETU BANDHASANA WITH BLOCKS AND A STRAP
BRIDGE POSE VARIATION

PROPS
- 1 nonskid mat
- 2 blankets
- 2 blocks
- 1 strap

This variation of Setu Bandhasana with Blocks and a Strap (Figure 5.17) helps to activate your kidneys.

Take two folded blankets and fold each of them in half lengthwise. Stack the blankets, one on top of the other, and place them crosswise on your nonskid mat. Then lie on your back with your shoulders at the clean edge of the blankets. Extend your arms by your sides with your palms facing down and broaden your shoulders. Bend your knees, place your feet flat on the floor in line with your sitting bones, and lift your pelvis.

Place one block flat on the floor under your pelvis, and stack the second block on its end. Position the blocks to support your lower sacrum and tailbone, not your upper sacrum. (If you cannot manage two blocks, use one block instead.) Then bring

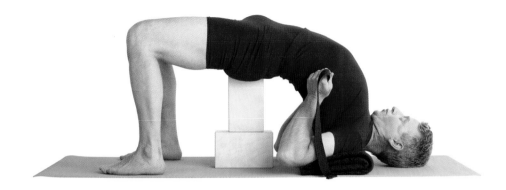

a strap across your lower back rib cage to support your kidneys. Hold the strap with your hands close to the sides of your rib cage and your elbows in line with the sides of your waist.

In Setu Bandhasana with Blocks and a Strap, relax your shoulders and widen your collarbones away from your sternal notch. Roll the inner corners of your collarbones toward your head, and move the outer corners of your collarbones toward your inner arms. At the same time, lengthen the back of your arms toward your elbows, and lift your shoulder blades toward your waist. Then press the strap firmly against your lower ribs, and lift your kidneys up and over the strap—like salmon leaping upstream. As your kidneys lift toward your lumbar spine, move your liver and stomach toward your inner groins to lengthen the front of your body. When you make this adjustment, your inner legs will feel stronger and will draw your thighbones together.

Hold this position for 1 to 2 minutes, maintaining the lift of your kidneys. Then release the strap, lift your pelvis, and remove the blocks. Rest your pelvis on the floor, with your knees bent and your head on the blankets. Allow your sacrum to relax before proceeding.

SALAMBA SARVANGASANA
SHOULDERSTAND

PROPS
• set up as determined in Chapter 1

In this variation of Salamba Sarvangasana (Figure 5.18), let the inner corners of your collarbones roll toward your head to bring you higher onto your shoulders.

Come into Salamba Sarvangasana as described in Chapter 1.

In Salamba Sarvangasana, place your hands flat on your back with your fingers pointing toward your waist and your lower rib cage resting lightly against your palms. Widen your collarbones away from your sternal notch, and soften the base of your throat. Let the inner corners of your collarbones roll gently toward your head as you lift your shoulder blades away from the blanket. At the same time, move the outer corners of your collarbones toward your inner arms, and lift your kidneys away from your hands evenly on your right and left sides. Then lift your inner groins away from your kidneys so that your legs balance evenly between your kidneys, at the back of your body, and your groins, at the front of your body.

Maintain this position for 3 to 10 minutes. Roll the inner corners of your collarbones toward your head, lift your kidneys away from your palms, and lift your inner groins away from your kidneys as you lengthen your legs. To come into Halasana (Figure 5.19), first, lengthen your kidneys; then draw your groins into your body as you lower your legs.

RELATED POSES. Salamba Sarvangasana variations

HALASANA
PLOUGH POSE

PROPS
• set up as determined in Chapter 1

5.19
Halasana

In this variation of Halasana (Figure 5.19), lift your inner groins away from your kidneys to lengthen and release your lumbar spine.

Come into Halasana from Salamba Sarvangasana (Figure 5.18).

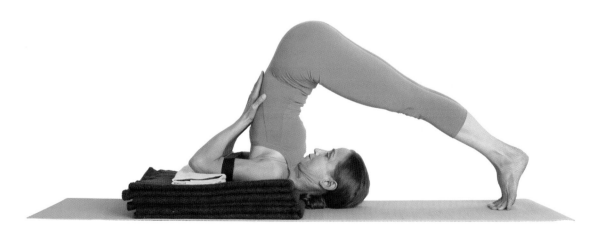

In Halasana, place your hands flat on your back with your fingers pointing toward your waist, and let your lower rib cage rest against your palms. Widen your collarbones away from your sternal notch, and soften the base of your throat. Lift your kidneys away from your thoracic spine so that your kidneys both lengthen and fill the palms of your hands. Then lift your groins away from your kidneys to activate your legs and release your lumbar spine. Move the base of your skull away from your sternal notch, and draw your eyes deeper into their sockets to relax your face.

Maintain this position quietly for 1 to 3 minutes, or about one-third the time you spent in Salamba Sarvangasana. Then release your hands from your back and roll out of the pose. Rest with your shoulders on the floor and your rib cage on the blankets.

5.20
Marichyasana III at the Wall

MARICHYASANA III AT THE WALL
POSE OF SAGE MARICHI III VARIATION

PROPS
- 1 nonskid mat
- 1 blanket
- 1 wall

OPTIONAL PROP
- 1 block

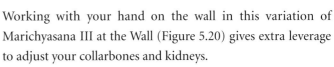

Working with your hand on the wall in this variation of Marichyasana III at the Wall (Figure 5.20) gives extra leverage to adjust your collarbones and kidneys.

Place your nonskid mat parallel to, and about 6 inches away from, a wall. Fold a blanket in half or in thirds, and lay it crosswise on the mat. Sit at the edge of the blanket with your legs extended and your right side facing the wall, 12 to 15 inches away from the wall. Bend your right leg and place your right foot flat on the floor in line with your right sitting bone. Turn your rib cage to face the wall, let your weight drop back onto your right hand, and turn your lower abdomen to the right. (Use a block under your right hand if you find it helpful.) Then bring your left arm over your right knee, and place your hand on the wall so that your left forearm forms a wedge between your right leg and the wall.

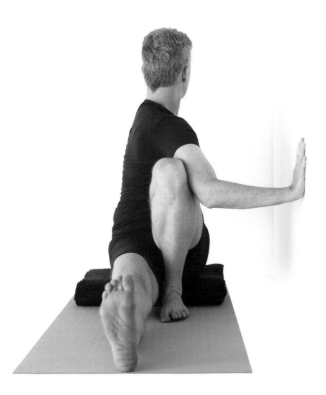

In Marichyasana III at the Wall, lift your left kidney away from your left inner groin, and turn it toward your lumbar spine. Then lift your right kidney away from your right inner groin, and turn it away from your thoracic spine. Relax your collarbones and widen your sternal notch. Roll the outer corner of your left collarbone down to bring your left shoulder forward, and lengthen your left collarbone toward your inner left arm. Roll the inner corner of your right collarbone up, and lengthen your right collarbone toward your inner right arm to open your right shoulder and move it back.

Maintain this position for about 1 minute. Use the leverage of your hand on the wall to help deepen the twist. Turn your left kidney toward your lumbar spine, and lift your right kidney toward your thoracic spine. Broaden your collarbones and lift your sternal notch as you turn your head to the right. Then roll your left collarbone down and your right collarbone up as you turn your manubrium to the right. Keep the back edge of your respiratory diaphragm broad. When you are ready, release your torso. Repeat to the other side.

RELATED POSES. Other sitting twists

PASCHIMOTTANASANA
SITTING FORWARD BEND

PROP
- 1 nonskid mat
- 1 blanket or wedge

OPTIONAL PROPS
- 1 strap

5.21
Paschimottanasana

In Paschimottanasana (Figure 5.21), first, roll the inner corners of your collarbones up to lengthen your arms and extend your spine as you come into the pose. Then roll the outer corners of your collarbones down to release your shoulder girdle as you move deeper into the forward bend.

Place a folded blanket or wedge on your nonskid mat. Then sit at the edge of the blanket or wedge with your legs extended and your hands by the sides of your pelvis. Draw your inner groins into your body, lift your kidneys toward your thoracic spine,

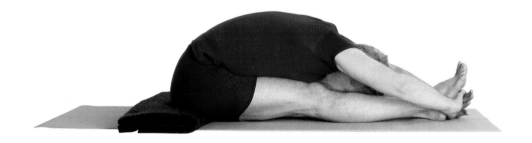

and widen your collarbones away from your sternal notch. With an inhalation, raise your arms overhead, rolling the inner corners of your collarbones up and lifting the outer corners of your collarbones as you lengthen your inner arms. With an exhalation, lengthen the back of your kidneys as you extend your torso over your thighs. Take hold of the soles of your feet with your hands. (Use a strap around your feet if you are less flexible).

In Paschimottanasana, draw your groins deep into your body, and lengthen the back of your kidneys toward your head. Turn the front of your kidneys toward your lumbar spine, so that your lower kidneys rest back against your lower ribs but your upper kidneys move deeper into your body. Then bend your elbows out to the side and widen your sternal notch. Roll the outer corners of your collarbones away from your head, and lengthen them toward your inner arms. Drop your chin toward your chest. Draw your eyes deep into their sockets, and release the base of your skull.

Hold this position for 1 to 2 minutes, exhaling softly from your kidneys. To come out of the pose, extend your arms forward with your palms facing each other. Then raise your head, roll the inner corners of your collarbones up, and lengthen from the outer corners of your collarbones toward your inner arms. With an inhalation, lift your arms overhead as you bring your torso upright. With an exhalation, lower your arms to the sides of your body.

Practice Notes. If you have a scoliosis or an imbalance in your lumbar area, one kidney may feel closer to your spine than the other. In this case, turn one kidney toward your spine and the other kidney away from your spine until they feel more equal. Remember to turn from your kidneys, not your diaphragm.

JANU SIRSASANA
HEAD-OF-THE-KNEE POSE

5.22
Janu Sirsasana

PROPS
- 1 nonskid mat
- 1 blanket or wedge

OPTIONAL PROPS
- 1 blanket or block
- 1 strap

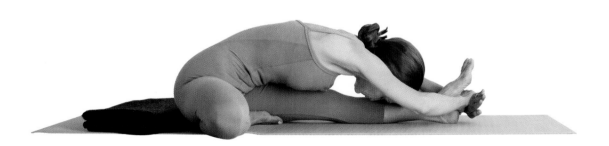

In this variation of Janu Sirsasana (Figure 5.22), first, let your collarbones roll toward your head to lengthen your spine actively as you come into the pose; then turn your collarbones away from your head to release into the forward bend.

Place a folded blanket or wedge on your nonskid mat. Then sit at the edge of the blanket or wedge with your legs extended. Place your right hand behind your right knee and bend your right leg. Draw your right heel toward your right groin, and rest the top of your right foot on the floor, with your knee out to the side. (If your right knee doesn't touch the floor, use a folded blanket or block for support.)

Place your hands on the floor by your outer hips, and broaden your collarbones away from the sternal notch to open your chest. Draw your left inner groin back into your body, and lift your right kidney away from your right inner groin. With an inhalation, raise your arms overhead, rolling your collarbones up and lifting the outer corners of your collarbones toward your inner arms. With an exhalation, lengthen the back of your kidneys as you extend your torso over your left thigh, and take hold of your left foot. If your hands reach beyond your foot, take hold of your left wrist with your right hand. (If your hamstrings are tight, hold your foot with a strap.)

In Janu Sirsasana, draw your left inner groin back into your body, and turn your left kidney away from your thoracic spine as you lengthen the left side of your rib cage. Broaden your right inner groin away from your pubic bone, and turn your right kidney toward your lumbar spine to bring your rib cage squarely over your extended leg. Then bend your elbows out to the side, and widen your sternal notch. Roll the outer corners of your collarbones away from your head, lengthening them toward your inner arms as you rest your forehead on your shin. Draw your eyes deep into their sockets, and release the base of your skull.

Hold this position for 1 to 2 minutes, exhaling softly from your kidneys. To come out of the pose, extend your arms forward with your palms facing each other. Then raise your head, roll your collarbones up, and lengthen from the outer corners of your collarbones toward your inner arms. With an inhalation, lift your arms overhead as you bring your torso upright. With an exhalation, lower your arms to the sides of your rib cage, extend your right leg, and repeat to the other side.

RELATED POSES. Other sitting forward bends

UJJAYI PRANAYAMA LYING
BASIC YOGA BREATHING

PROPS

- 1 nonskid mat
- 2 blankets
- 1 facecloth

This variation of Ujjayi Pranayama Lying (Figure 5.23) increases awareness of the kidneys.

Fold one blanket in half lengthwise, and place it on your mat to support your rib cage. When folded, this blanket should measure about 8 inches wide and 30 inches long. Fold a second blanket in half or in thirds crosswise, and place it at the top end of your first blanket to support your neck and head. Place a facecloth, folded in quarters to form a long, narrow strip about 3 inches wide, at the bottom edge of your first blanket to support your lower rib cage and kidneys.

Then lie on your back, and adjust the height and placement of your props, as necessary. Check that the first blanket supports your lower ribs but not your waist or pelvis, and that the second blanket supports the base of your skull and your neck, so that your chin is slightly tucked. Make sure that the folded facecloth fits comfortably into the triangular space between your lower rib cage and the bottom edge of your first blanket, so that your kidneys rest on a firm surface. Then lie quietly for 1 to 2 minutes, releasing the weight of your arms and legs with each exhalation.

Begin your breathing practice with a deep, soft exhalation. With a deep, soft inhalation, direct your incoming breath toward your kidneys, and let the sides of your rib cage gently expand. Your kidneys should feel broad and firm as they come into closer contact with your blanket. With a deep exhalation, keep the sides of your rib cage lifted, and let your breath release from the center of your kidneys. Toward the end of the exhalation, gently turn the front edges of your liver and stomach toward your navel to deepen the movement of the out breath.

Repeat this cycle for 3 to 5 minutes. Let each inhalation and each exhalation build naturally. Focus on the movement of your kidneys. Feel their expansiveness. Be more concerned with the quality and rhythm of your breath than with the volume of your breath. When you are finished, rest for another minute until your breath has returned to normal; then turn onto your side and sit up.

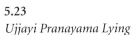

5.23
Ujjayi Pranayama Lying

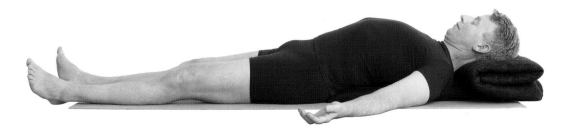

UJJAYI PRANAYAMA SITTING
BASIC YOGA BREATHING

PROPS
- 1 nonskid mat
- 1 blanket

OPTIONAL PROPS
- 1 or 2 blocks or blankets
- 1 wedge

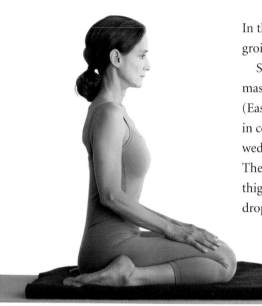

In this variation of Ujjayi Pranayama Sitting, lift your kidneys away from your inner groins, and widen your collarbones to prolong your inhalation.

Sit at the edge of a folded blanket in your most comfortable sitting position: Padmasana (Lotus Pose, Figure 3.21), Siddhasana (Perfect Pose, Figure 4.23), Sukhasana (Easy Pose, Figure 6.22), or Virasana (Hero Pose, Figure 5.24). If your knees are not in contact with the floor, use blocks or blankets to support them. (You can also use a wedge under your sitting bones to give an additional lift to your pelvis and spine.) Then bring your elbows to the sides of your waist, and place your hands on your thighs with your palms down. Close your eyes gently, widen your collarbones, and drop your chin toward your sternal notch.

above:
5.24
Virasana

below:
5.25
Savasana

Begin with a deep, soft exhalation. With a deep inhalation, lift your kidneys away from your inner groins. At the same time, roll the inner corners of your collarbones toward your head and deepen your sternal notch. Widen the outer corners of your collarbones and lengthen your inner arms. At the end of the inhalation, stabilize your rib cage and exhale slowly from the center of your kidneys. Repeat this cycle for 3 to 5 minutes. Then let your breath return to normal, raise your head, and change the cross of your legs. Repeat for another 3 to 5 minutes. Then rest in Savasana (Figure 5.25).

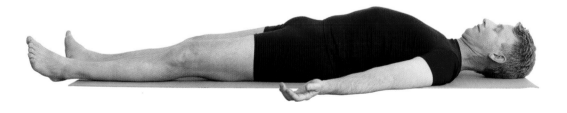

SAVASANA
RELAXATION POSE

PROP	OPTIONAL PROP
• 1 nonskid mat	• 1 blanket

This variation of Savasana (Figure 5.25) brings your awareness to your kidneys and groins.

Lie on your back on a nonskid mat, with your knees bent and your feet on the floor in line with your sitting bones. (If the base of your skull feels tight, place a folded blanket under your head and neck.) Bend your elbows and press the back of your upper arms into the floor. Keep equal weight on your inner and outer elbows as you straighten your arms and rest the back of your hands on the floor. Then press your sacrum into the floor, and extend your legs, one at a time. Relax your pelvis and knees, and allow your legs to roll out.

Close your eyes and soften your inward gaze. With each inhalation, direct your breath toward your inner groins. With each exhalation, breathe out from your kidneys. Continue with this Savasana for 5 to 8 minutes. As your groins relax and your kidneys sink into the floor, the pause at the end of exhalation grows deeper and longer.

When you feel rested, bend your knees and turn onto your side before sitting up.

▶
PRACTICE SEQUENCE (READ DOWN)

TADASANA	SALABHASANA	MARICHYASANA III AT THE WALL
ADHO MUKHA SVANASANA	URDHVA DHANURASANA	
UTTHITA TRIKONASANA	PARIVRTTA UTTANASANA	PASCHIMOTTANASANA
PADANGUSTHASANA	SALAMBA SIRSASANA	JANU SIRSASANA
VIRABHADRASANA I	SETU BANDHASANA WITH BLOCKS AND A STRAP	UJJAYI PRANAYAMA LYING
UTTANASANA		UJJAYI PRANAYAMA SITTING
PARIVRTTA TRIKONASANA	SALAMBA SARVANGASANA	SAVASANA
PINCHA MAYURASANA AT THE WALL	HALASANA	

6 ALIGN YOUR SHOULDER BLADES

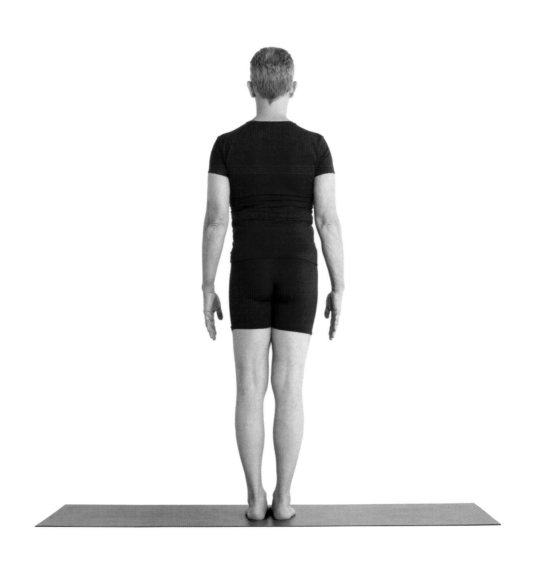

THE SHOULDER BLADES (scapulae) are flat, triangular bones that hang vertically on the surface of your upper back rib cage. They are attached to the outer corners of your collarbones via the acromion process—the knobby protrusion that you can feel along the outer ridge of your shoulder, and form part of the shoulder girdle. In Tadasana (Figure 6.5), the inner edges of your shoulder blades (known anatomically as medial borders) lie parallel to your spine; the top edges (or superior borders) are parallel to your shoulders; and the outer edges (or lateral borders) rest against the sides of your rib cage (Figure 6.1).

The shoulder blades have three corners (or angles) as well as three edges. In Tadasana, the bottom tip (or inferior angle) of your shoulder blade points down toward the floor; the inner corner of the top edge (or superior angle) points toward the base of your neck; and the outer corner (or lateral angle) points toward your upper arm. The outer corner of your shoulder blade forms a depression called the glenoid cavity that articulates with the head of your upper arm bone (humerus), and is thus a part of your shoulder joint.

When you stand in Tadasana, ideally, your shoulder blades rest flat against your back rib cage, with the inner edges, outer edges, and top edges all touching evenly. When you raise your arms out to the side, lift them overhead, or extend them behind your back, your shoulder blades should follow and adjust to the contours of your rib cage. If you can maintain even contact of your shoulder blades throughout their range of movement, you are, in effect, balancing the muscles that stabilize and protect your shoulder joints and preventing shoulder injury.

Your shoulder blades have a dual function: they must respond easily to the movement of your arms in order to coordinate and sustain the complex actions of your shoulder joints; and they must also support your back rib cage in a way that strengthens the broad muscles of your upper back. If your shoulder blades grip your rib cage too tightly, their freedom of movement will be restricted. If your shoulder blades hang too loosely, your upper back does not support the weight of your arms. Find the place where your shoulder blades rest snugly against your rib cage without gripping.

When adjusting your shoulder blades, you may find it helpful to think of three separate phases. These three steps can be applied to every pose. Step 1: Relax your shoulders and widen the top edges of your shoulder blades away from your spine. Step 2:

6.1

Shoulder Blades

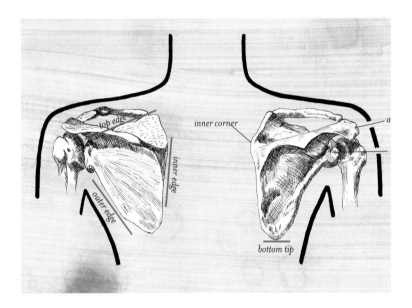

ROUND RIB CAGE WITH
SHOULDER BLADES TILTING
FORWARD AND UP

SQUARE RIB CAGE WITH
SHOULDER BLADES TILTING
BACK AND DOWN

NEUTRAL RIB CAGE WITH
SHOULDER BLADES
VERTICAL

Align your shoulder blades vertically so that the top edges and bottom tips contact your rib cage evenly. Step 3: Align your shoulder blades laterally so that the inner edges and outer edges contact your rib cage evenly.

Step 1. When adjusting your shoulder blades, first of all, relax your shoulders and release the top edges of your shoulder blades away from your spine. Especially in Adho Mukha Svanasana (Figure 6.6) and Salamba Sirsasana (Figure 6.17), do not use your arms to pull your shoulder blades apart, but let them release gently away from your spine. Move from the core of your body outward. Likewise in Tadasana, do not use your shoulders to pull your shoulder blades down your back. When you relax your shoulders and widen the top edges of your shoulder blades, your shoulder blades naturally drop away from the grip of your shoulder muscles (trapezius).

Step 2. Once you have widened the top edges of your shoulder blades away from your spine, check that your shoulder blades are vertically aligned with your upper back. When aligned vertically, the top edges and the bottom tips of your shoulder blades are parallel to and equidistant from the back of your rib cage. In this balanced state, your shoulder blades and your rib cage rest easily against each other.

If the bottom tips of your shoulder blades press into your rib cage and the top edges pull away in Tadasana or any other pose, you are overarching your back, and causing your floating ribs to protrude at the front of your body. This happens especially in Adho Mukha Svanasana and Salamba Sirsasana. In this case, first widen your shoulder blades; then press the top edges of your shoulder blades toward your rib cage and release the bottom tips away from your rib cage, so that your shoulder blades lie parallel with your upper back.

On the other hand, if the top edges of your shoulder blades press onto your rib cage and the bottom tips pull away, you are rounding your upper back and collapsing your xiphoid process. This happens frequently in Urdhva Mukha Svanasana (Figure 4.12) and Salamba Sarvangasana (Figure 6.18). In this case, draw the top edges of your shoulder blades away from your rib cage, and lift the bottom tips of your shoulder blades toward your rib cage, so that your shoulder blades are once again parallel with your upper back.

Step 3. Once you have aligned your shoulder blades vertically, adjust your shoulder blades laterally, so that the inner edges and the outer edges of your shoulder blades come into even contact with your rib cage. If you tend to round your upper back, the outer edges of your shoulder blades are drawn forward, and the inner edges turn away from your upper back. If you tend to flatten your thoracic spine, the inner edges of your shoulder blades press forward, but the outer edges are pulled back. In a balanced position, the inner edges and the outer edges of your shoulder blades hug your rib cage evenly.

When adjusting your shoulder blades laterally, take your body type into account: identify whether the shape of your rib cage is round, flat, or somewhere in between. If your rib cage is round, your chest is deep from front to back, your thoracic spine is overly rounded, and the front edge of your respiratory diaphragm tends to be tight and narrow. If your rib cage is flat, or rectangular, your chest is shallow from front to back, your thoracic spine is overly flattened, and the front edge of your respiratory diaphragm is generally loose and broad (Figure 6.2).

The shape of your rib cage influences the resting position of your shoulder blades in Tadasana. If your rib cage is round, the outer edges of your shoulder blades are drawn forward, and the muscles of the side chest that hold them in place (teres major, teres minor, and anterior serratus) are thick and foreshortened. At the same time, the inner edges of your shoulder blades pull away from your spine, overly stretching the muscles of your upper back. In my experience, the wider the space between the inner edges of your shoulder blades, the weaker your upper back.

If your rib cage is round, focus on the inner edges of your shoulder blades when you stand in Tadasana. First, lift your kidneys away from your inner groins; then lift the inner edges of your shoulder blades away from your kidneys. Feel how this adjustment activates your rhomboids (the muscles that draw the inner edges of your shoulder blades toward your spine) and strengthens your whole upper back! At the same time, draw the outer edges of your shoulder blades back and down, and lengthen the sides of your chest. The inner and outer edges of your shoulder blades should now rest evenly against your rib cage.

If your rib cage is rectangular, the inner edges of your shoulder blades tend to grip your midthoracic vertebrae like pincers, flattening your upper spine, narrowing your upper back, and thrusting your midsternum forward. At the same time, there is a significant gap between the outer edges of your shoulder blades and the sides of your rib cage. The muscles that draw the outer edges of your shoulder blades toward your rib cage (teres minor and anterior serratus) are lax and loose, and the flesh of your back armpits is thick and slack.

If your rib cage is rectangular, focus on the outer edges of your shoulder blades. To adjust your shoulder blades in Tadasana, start by widening your midsternum. (If you keep your midsternum soft and broad, your shoulder blades will not pinch your midthoracic spine). Then gently squeeze your back armpits, and bring the outer edges of your shoulder blades into firm contact with the sides of your chest. At the same

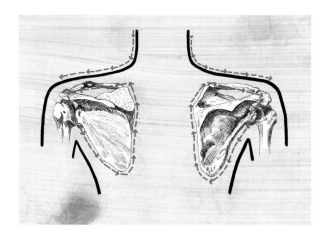 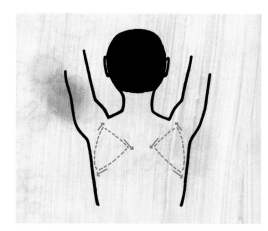

left:
6.3
*Circular Movement
of the Shoulder Blades
in Tadasana*

right:
6.4
*Circular Movement of the
Shoulder Blades Reversed,
Arms Overhead*

time, widen the top edges of your shoulder blades away from your spine, and lift the inner edges of your shoulder blades away from your kidneys. Feel how the inner edges and outer edges of your shoulder blades now rest evenly against your rib cage.

A word about armpits. In this book, I refer to front armpits and back armpits; I also mention inner armpits and outer armpits. When you stand in Tadasana, your front armpits are at the front of your body, and your back armpits at the back of your body. When you raise your arms overhead, your front armpits are closer to the median line of your body, so I refer to them as inner armpits. Your back armpits are farther away from the median line, so I call them outer armpits. In other words, your front armpits become your inner armpits, and your back armpits become your outer armpits as your arms change position.

The practice sequence in this chapter emphasizes the circular movement of your shoulder blades to strengthen and broaden your upper back, give support to your head and neck, and mobilize your shoulder joints. When you stand in Tadasana, imagine a circular action that follows the edges of your shoulder blades. Lift the inner edges of your shoulder blades away from your kidneys, release the top edges away from your spine, and draw the outer edges down toward your kidneys. This adjustment strengthens your upper back without gripping or hardening your midthoracic spine (Figure 6.3).

As the top edges of your shoulder blades release away from your spine, the inner corners lift up to support the base of your neck, the outer corners descend to widen your shoulders, and the bottom tips move closer to your spine without pressing forward.

When you raise your arms overhead, as in Urdhva Hastasana I (Figure 7.6), the circular action should be reversed. Move the inner edges of your shoulder blades away from the base of your neck, lengthen the outer edges up toward your arms, and draw the top edges in toward the base of your neck. This adjustment widens your upper back without hunching your shoulders (Figure 6.4).

As the inner edges of your shoulder blades move away from the base of your neck, lift the outer corners toward your arms to create space in your shoulder joints, draw the inner corners away from the back of your head to release the base of your neck, and move the bottom tips away from your midthoracic spine without letting them press forward.

The following practice sequence focuses on the alignment and movement of your shoulder blades.

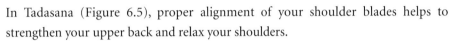

TADASANA
MOUNTAIN POSE

PROP
- 1 nonskid mat

6.5
Tadasana

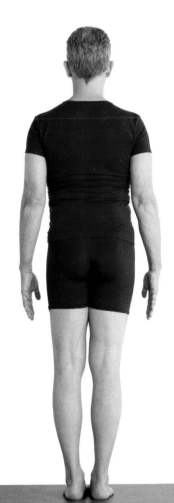

In Tadasana (Figure 6.5), proper alignment of your shoulder blades helps to strengthen your upper back and relax your shoulders.

Stand on your mat in Tadasana with your feet together and your arms by your sides. Bring the center of your perineum in line with the crown of your head to adjust your pelvis. Relax your shoulders and widen your collarbones away from your sternal notch. Move the top edges of your shoulder blades away from your spine, and let them release away from the ridge of your shoulders without deliberately pulling them down.

Then widen your midsternum and lift the inner edges of your shoulder blades away from your kidneys. Let the top edges of your shoulder blades release away from your spine, but move the bottom tips of your shoulder blades toward your spine. Firm the muscles of your back armpits, and press the outer edges of your shoulder blades against the sides of your rib cage. Draw the outer edges of your shoulder blades down toward your kidneys, without gripping your midthoracic spine.

Remain in Tadasana for another 30 seconds, deepening your awareness of the circular movement of your shoulder blades. Let the inner corners of your shoulder blades lift up to lengthen your neck. Allow the outer corners of your shoulder blades to descend to release your shoulders. Let the bottom tips of your shoulder blades move gently toward your spine, without pressing forward. Return to this position between each of the standing poses to readjust your shoulder blades and strengthen your upper back.

ADHO MUKHA SVANASANA
DOWNWARD-FACING DOG POSE

PROP

• 1 nonskid mat

In this variation of Adho Mukha Svanasana (Figure 6.6), the top edges, inner edges, and outer edges of the shoulder blades are all aligned with the contours of your rib cage.

Start in a kneeling position with your hands on the floor slightly in front of your shoulders and with your pelvis over your knees. With an inhalation, press the back of your rib cage against your shoulder blades so that your upper back is rounded, and lengthen the top edges of your shoulder blades away from your spine. With an exhalation, turn your toes under and lift your pelvis as you straighten your legs.

In Adho Mukha Svanasana, lift your inner groins into your body and lengthen your kidneys. Press the top edges of your shoulder blades against your upper rib cage, and lift the bottom tips of your shoulder blades away from your lower rib cage so that your shoulder blades lie parallel with your upper back. When your shoulder blades are vertically aligned, lift the inner corners of your shoulder blades away from your neck, lengthen down through your arms from the outer corners, and move the bottom tips of your shoulder blades away from your spine to widen your upper back.

Maintain this position for 1 to 2 minutes. With an inhalation, relax and widen the top edges of your shoulder blades. With an exhalation, lengthen your outer arms from the center of your outer armpits, and turn the outer edges of your shoulder

6.6
Adho Mukha Svanasana

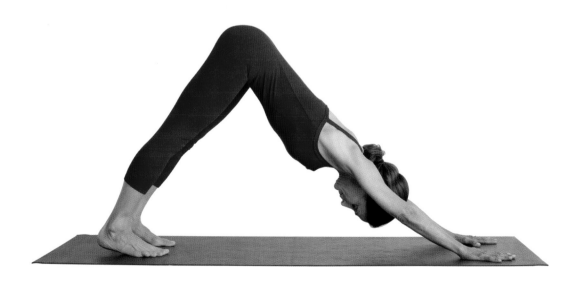

blades toward your rib cage as you lengthen the sides of your chest. Balance your rib cage evenly between your outer shoulder blades on your right and left sides. To come out of the pose, bend your knees and rest in Adho Mukha Virasana (Child's Pose, Figure 3.11b).

6.7
Utthita Trikonasana

UTTHITA TRIKONASANA
EXTENDED TRIANGLE POSE

PROP
• 1 nonskid mat

OPTIONAL PROP
• 1 block

In this variation of Utthita Trikonasana (Figure 6.7), the shoulder blades help to strengthen the upper back and open the rib cage.

Stand on your mat in Tadasana (Figure 6.5), and separate your legs so that your feet are 4 to 4½ feet apart. Turn your left foot in 30 degrees and your right foot out 90 degrees. Bring the center of your perineum in line with the center of your respiratory diaphragm and lengthen your spine. With an inhalation, widen your midsternum and raise your arms to shoulder level. Release the top edges of your shoulder blades away from your spine, and move the bottom tips of your shoulder blades toward your spine. With an exhalation, extend your torso over your right leg. Bring your right hand to the floor by your outer right ankle. (Use a block under your hand if you cannot reach the floor easily.)

In Utthita Trikonasana, check that the center of your perineum is in line with the center of your respiratory diaphragm. Then widen your midsternum and lengthen your spine. To bring your right shoulder in line with your right leg, move the bottom tip of your right shoulder blade toward your spine, and lengthen the top edge of your right shoulder blade away from your spine. To deepen the twist, lift your torso away from your outer right armpit, and press the outer edge of your right shoulder blade against your rib cage. To bring your left shoulder in line with the left side of your rib cage, lift the bottom tip of your left shoulder blade away from your spine, and lengthen your outer left armpit. At the same time, move the inner corner of your left shoulder blade away from the back of your head to release your neck.

Maintain this position for 1 minute. Let the bottom tip of your right shoulder blade move toward the spine, and the bottom tip of your left shoulder blade move away from the spine. To come out of the pose, stabilize your right shoulder blade, and lift up from your left shoulder blade. Then repeat to the other side.

Practice Notes. In asymmetrical poses, move the bottom tip of one shoulder blade toward your spine to strengthen your upper back on one side, while you move the bottom tip of the other shoulder blade laterally away from your spine to widen your upper back on the other side. In Utthita Trikonasana to the right, move the bottom tip of your right shoulder blade toward your spine to firm the right side of your rib cage and bring it forward. At the same time, with your left arm raised, release the bottom tip of your left shoulder blade away from your spine to widen the left side of your rib cage and draw it back.

RELATED POSES. Utthita Parsvakonasana, Virabhadrasana II, Ardha Chandrasana

UTTANASANA
STANDING FORWARD BEND

PROP
• 1 nonskid mat

OPTIONAL PROP
• 1 block

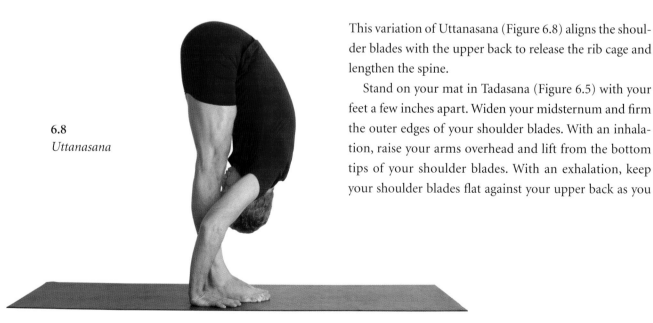

6.8
Uttanasana

This variation of Uttanasana (Figure 6.8) aligns the shoulder blades with the upper back to release the rib cage and lengthen the spine.

Stand on your mat in Tadasana (Figure 6.5) with your feet a few inches apart. Widen your midsternum and firm the outer edges of your shoulder blades. With an inhalation, raise your arms overhead and lift from the bottom tips of your shoulder blades. With an exhalation, keep your shoulder blades flat against your upper back as you extend your torso forward. Place your hands on the floor by the sides of your feet, with your elbows in line with your shoulders. (Use a block under your hands if they do not reach the floor easily.)

In Uttanasana, release the top edges of your shoulder blades away from your spine, and lengthen from the outer corners of your shoulder blades to your inner elbows. To deepen your forward bend, lift the bottom tips of your shoulder blades away from your lower rib cage, and press the top edges of your shoulder blades against your upper back. At the same time, lengthen from the center of your outer armpits to your inner elbows, and firm the outer edges of your shoulder blades against the sides of your rib cage.

Remain in Uttanasana for 1 minute. With an inhalation, allow the sides of your chest to lengthen. With an exhalation, turn the outer edges of your shoulder blades toward your rib cage. Let your rib cage balance evenly between your outer right shoulder blade and your outer left shoulder blade, like a wicker basket between two strong handles.

To come out of Uttanasana, place your hands on your hips, press your shoulder blades flat against your upper back, and, with an inhalation, lift your torso. With an exhalation, return to Tadasana.

RELATED POSE. Prasarita Padottanasana (Phase 2)

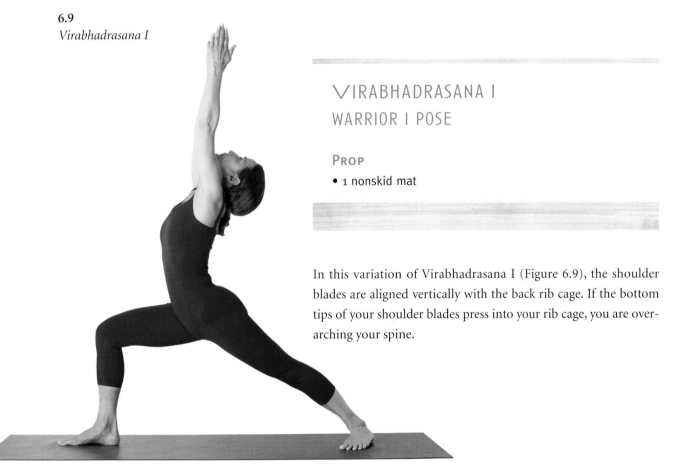

6.9
Virabhadrasana I

VIRABHADRASANA I
WARRIOR I POSE

PROP
• 1 nonskid mat

In this variation of Virabhadrasana I (Figure 6.9), the shoulder blades are aligned vertically with the back rib cage. If the bottom tips of your shoulder blades press into your rib cage, you are overarching your spine.

Stand on your mat in Tadasana (Figure 6.5), and separate your legs about 3½ feet apart. Turn your right foot out 90 degrees and your left foot in 60 degrees. Draw your right groin back into your body, and turn your left groin toward the median line of your body, so that your pelvis directly faces your right leg. Then place your hands on your hips with your thumbs pressing down at the top edge of your sacrum. Lift your kidneys away from your inner groins, and lift the inner edges of your shoulder blades away from your kidneys. Widen the top edges of your shoulder blades away from your spine, and let your head drop back, but only if it feels comfortable on your neck. (If you have any problems with your neck, keep your head erect.) With an inhalation, raise your arms overhead with your palms facing each other, and lift from the bottom tips of your shoulder blades. With an exhalation, bend your right knee to form a right angle.

In Virabhadrasana I, first check that your shoulder blades are vertically aligned. If the bottom tips of your shoulder blades press forward, let them release away from your lower rib cage and broaden your midsternum. Then turn the outer edge of your left shoulder blade toward your rib cage to bring the sides of your rib cage level. Draw the inner corners of your shoulder blades away from your neck, and lift your arms from the outer corners of your shoulder blades.

Maintain this position for 30 seconds. Relax your shoulder blades, so that they are not gripping your back rib cage. Lift your arms from the space between your shoulder blades and your rib cage. Balance your rib cage evenly between your outer shoulder blades, and relax your head and neck.

To come out of the pose, inhale as you straighten your right leg; exhale as you lower your arms. Repeat to the other side.

PADANGUSTHASANA
TOE-HOLDING POSE

PROP
• 1 nonskid mat

OPTIONAL PROP
• 1 block

In the first phase of Padangusthasana (Figure 6.10a), your arms are fully extended, your head is lifted, and your spine assumes a gentle backbend. In the second phase (Figure 6.10b), your elbows are bent, your head hangs freely, and your spine releases into a forward bend.

Phase 1. Stand on your mat in Tadasana (Figure 6.5) with your feet a few inches apart, and place your hands on your hips. With an inhalation, widen your midsternum, lift the inner edges of your shoulder blades away from your kidneys, and let your head drop back. At the same time, lengthen from the center of your back armpits toward your inner elbows, and firm the outer edges of your shoulder blades against the sides of your chest. With an exhalation, keep your shoulder blades in firm contact with your rib cage as you lengthen your torso forward.

When your torso is parallel to the floor, extend your arms and wrap your second and third fingers around your big toes. (If you cannot reach the floor without rounding your upper back, use a block under your hands.) Let the bottom tips of your shoulder blades move toward each other to lengthen your thoracic spine. Lift the inner corners of your shoulder blades toward the base of your neck to release your cervical spine. Maintain this position for several breaths.

Phase 2. Now bend your elbows out to the side, bring your midsternum toward your legs, and release your head and neck. Press the top edges of your shoulder blades against your rib cage to deepen the forward bend; lengthen from the outer corners of your shoulder blades toward your inner elbows to widen your upper back. Maintain this position for several breaths. To come out of the pose, extend your arms, lift your head, and draw the bottom tips of your shoulder blades toward your spine. With an inhalation, lengthen your spine. With an exhalation, return to Tadasana.

RELATED POSE. Prasarita Padottanasana

6.10a
Padangusthasana, Phase 1

6.10b
Padangusthasana, Phase 2

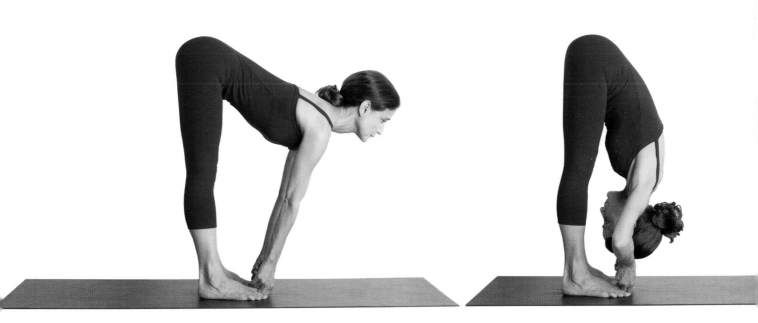

PARIVRTTA TRIKONASANA
REVOLVED TRIANGLE POSE

PROP
- 1 nonskid mat

OPTIONAL PROP
- 1 block

6.11
Parivrtta Trikonasana

In this variation of Parivrtta Trikonasana (Figure 6.11), the movement of your shoulder blades helps to strengthen your upper back and deepen the twist.

Start in Tadasana (Figure 6.5), and separate your legs about 3½ feet apart. Turn your left foot in about 60 degrees and your right foot out 90 degrees. Then place your hands on your hips, and turn your pelvis to face your right leg. Draw your right inner groin back into your body, and widen your left inner groin to bring your hips level. With an inhalation, turn your midsternum to face your right thigh, and raise your left arm overhead. Firm the outer edge of your left shoulder blade, and lengthen the left side of your chest. With an exhalation, turn from the outer edge of your left shoulder blade, and extend your torso forward over your right leg. Place your left hand by your

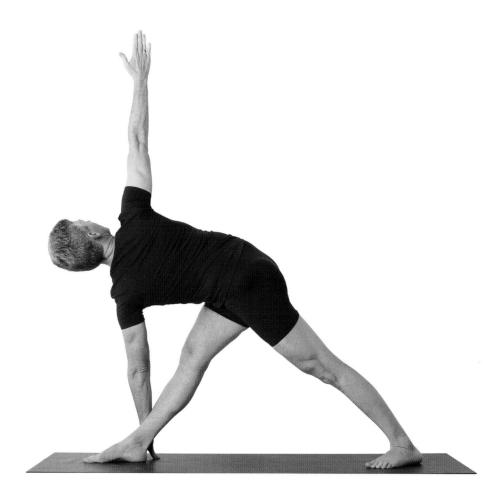

outer right ankle, and raise your right arm toward the ceiling. (If you are less flexible, place your left hand by your inner right ankle. Use a block under your hand, if necessary. Ideally, your spine should be parallel to the floor.)

In Parivrtta Trikonasana, bring the center of your perineum in line with the center of your respiratory diaphragm and lengthen your spine. To bring your left shoulder in line with your right ankle, move the bottom tip of your left shoulder blade toward the spine, and lengthen the top edge away from the spine. To deepen the twist, firm the outer edge of your left shoulder blade, and lift your rib cage away from your left back armpit. To bring your right shoulder in line with the right side of your rib cage, lift the bottom tip of your right shoulder blade away from the spine, and lengthen your outer right armpit. At the same time, move the inner corner of your right shoulder blade away from the back of your head to release your neck.

Maintain this position for 30 seconds. Let the bottom tip of your left shoulder blade move toward the spine, and the bottom tip of your right shoulder blade move away from the spine. To come out of the pose, stabilize your left shoulder blade, and lift up from your right shoulder blade. Then repeat to the other side.

RELATED POSE. Parivrtta Ardha Chandrasana

6.12
Pincha Mayurasana at the Wall

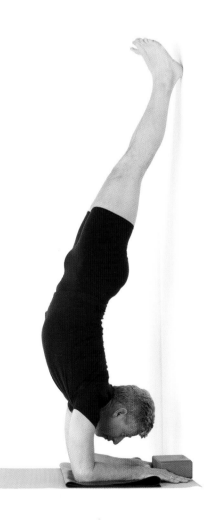

PINCHA MAYURASANA AT THE WALL
ELBOW BALANCE

PROPS
- 1 nonskid mat
- 1 wall
- 1 block

In this variation of Pincha Mayurasana at the Wall (Figure 6.12), the bottom tips of your shoulder blades move away from the spine to widen your upper back and release your thoracic spine.

Lay a nonskid mat folded in half or in quarters at the base of a wall. Place a block flat on the mat with its longest side against the wall to separate and stabilize your hands. Kneel in front of the mat, and position your hands so that your index fingers touch the sides of the block, your thumbs press the front edge of the block, and your palms lie flat.

Now rest the back of your rib cage against your shoulder blades so that your upper back is rounded, and widen the top edges of your shoulder blades away from your spine. Then turn your toes under, and lift your pelvis to straighten your legs. With an inhalation, bend one leg and step the foot a few inches closer to the wall. With an exhalation, keep your other leg straight as you swing it in a wide arc toward the wall. Let the momentum of your straight leg draw your bent leg away from the floor. Rest your heels on the wall with your legs extended; then lengthen the sides of your chest.

In Pincha Mayurasana at the Wall, press the top edges of your shoulder blades against your upper back, and lift the bottom tips of your shoulder blades away from your lower ribs so that your lumbar spine can lengthen. Then move the bottom tips of your shoulder blades away from your spine laterally to widen your upper back and release your thoracic spine. At the same time, draw the inner corners of your shoulder blades away from the base of your neck to lengthen your cervical spine and lift your head.

Maintain this position for another 30 seconds. With an inhalation, lift the bottom tips of your shoulder blades away from your lower rib cage, and lengthen the sides of your chest. With an exhalation, lengthen down from the center of your outer armpits, and turn the outer edges of your shoulder blades toward your rib cage. To come out of the pose, keep the inner corners of your shoulder blades lifted, release your inner groins, and lower your legs. Rest for several breaths in Adho Mukha Virasana (Child's Pose, Figure 3.11b).

RELATED POSE. Adho Mukha Vrksasana

USTRASANA
CAMEL POSE

PROPS
- 1 nonskid mat
- 1 blanket

OPTIONAL PROPS
- 1 block
- 1 bolster

6.13
Ustrasana

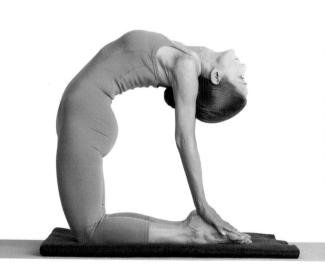

In this variation of Ustrasana (Figure 6.13), lift the bottom tips of your shoulder blades toward your lower ribs, and move the top edges away from your upper back to bring your shoulder blades parallel to your back rib cage.

Start in a kneeling position on a folded blanket, with your knees a few inches apart. (Place a block lengthwise between your feet if they tend to slide together.) Put your hands on your outer hips, and draw your elbows back so that your upper arms are parallel. Then widen your mid-sternum and firm the outer edges of your shoulder blades. With an inhalation, lift your kidneys away from your inner groins, and lift the inner edges of your shoulder blades away from your kidneys. Let your head drop back, but only if it feels comfortable on your neck. (If you have neck problems, keep your head lifted and tuck your chin toward your sternum). With an exhalation, lift the sides of your chest away from your back armpits, as you extend your arms and place your hands on your heels. (If you cannot reach your feet easily, place a bolster crosswise on your lower calves to support your hands.)

In Ustrasana, lift the bottom tips of your shoulder blades toward your lower ribs, and draw the top edges away from your upper back so that your shoulder blades lie parallel with the back of your rib cage. Then gently widen your midsternum, firm your back armpits, and press the outer edges of your shoulder blades against the sides of your rib cage.

Remain in Ustrasana for another 30 seconds. With an inhalation, lift the bottom tips of your shoulder blades toward your lower ribs to open your chest. With an exhalation, widen your midsternum and draw the top edges of your shoulder blades away from your upper back to release the base of your neck. To come out of the pose, inhale as you lift from the inner edges of your shoulder blades; exhale as you sit back on your heels. Repeat two or three times.

RELATED POSES. Urhdva Mukha Svanasana, Salabhasana, other backbends

URDHVA HASTASANA II
SUPINE MOUNTAIN POSE WITH ARMS OVERHEAD

PROPS
- 1 nonskid mat
- 1 wedge

- 1 strap

OPTIONAL PROP
- 1 blanket

6.14a
Urdhva Hastasana II,
Phase 1

This variation of Urdhva Hastasana II, consisting of three phases, requires a strap to hold your arms in place and a wedge to support your rib cage or shoulder blades.

Phase 1. Lie on your back with your knees bent and your feet flat on the floor. Lift your pelvis and place a wedge under your lower ribcage with the thick edge supporting your floating ribs and the thin edge pointing toward your shoulders (Figure 6.14a).

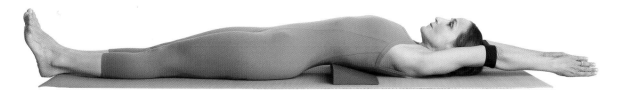

Make a loop with your strap approximately 8 to 10 inches in diameter, and place it on your upper arms just above your elbows. Then extend your legs, raise your arms overhead, and rest them on the floor. (If your arms do not reach the floor, use a folded blanket for support.) Bring your awareness to the back of your body. With an inhalation, broaden your floating ribs against the wedge, and lengthen the sides of your chest. With an exhalation, release your breath from the center of your kidneys. Repeat for three to six cycles of breath; then lower your arms.

Phase 2. For this phase, move the wedge a few inches higher, so that the thick edge of the wedge supports the bottom tips of your shoulder blades and the thin edge points toward your shoulders (Figure 6.14a). Readjust the belt above your elbows and raise your arms overhead. Relax your shoulders and upper back. With an inhalation, broaden your shoulder blades against the wedge, and lengthen your inner arms. With an exhalation, widen your midthoracic vertebrae. Repeat for three to six cycles of breath; then lower your arms.

6.14b
Urdhva Hastasana II, Phase 2

6.14c
Urdhva Hastasana II, Phase 3

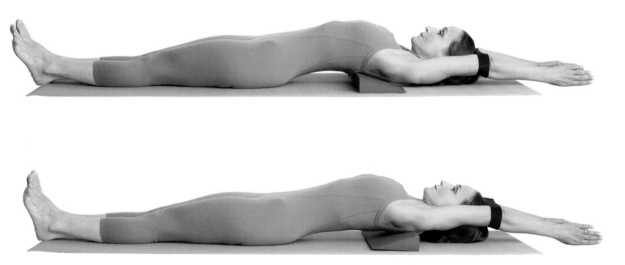

Phase 3. Now turn the wedge and move it 1 or 2 inches higher, so that the thick edge of the wedge supports the top edges of your shoulder blades, and the thin edge points toward your waist (Figure 6.14c). Readjust the belt above your elbows, raise your arms overhead, and extend your legs. With an inhalation, widen the top edges of your shoulder blades and lengthen your outer armpits. With an exhalation, relax your upper back against the wedge and release your arms. Feel the openness of your shoulder joints. Repeat for three to six cycles of breath. Then lower your arms, remove the belt, bend your knees, and turn onto your side.

Practice Notes. Urdhva Hastasana II releases tightness in your upper back, facilitates the movement of your shoulder blades, and frees your shoulder joints. It is an effective preparation for inverted poses, such as Adho Mukha Vrksasana at the Wall (Figure 3.11a), Pincha Mayurasana at the Wall (Figure 6.12), and Salamba Sirsasana (Figure 6.17), and for backbends where your arms are raised overhead, such as Urdhva Dhanurasana (Figure 6.15) and Viparita Dandasana with Feet on a Chair (Figure 8.17).

URDHVA DHANURASANA
UPWARD-FACING BOW POSE

PROP

• 1 nonskid mat

In Urdhva Dhanurasana (Figure 6.15), lift up from the bottom tips of your shoulder blades so that your shoulder blades are vertically aligned with your back rib cage.

Lie on your back on a nonskid mat. Then bend your knees and place your feet on the floor in line with your sitting bones and 2 to 3 inches away. Make sure that your feet point directly forward and do not turn out. Bring your arms overhead and place your palms on the floor in line with your shoulders so that your upper arms are parallel to each other. Then widen your shoulders and relax your shoulder blades. With an inhalation, lengthen from the bottom tips of your shoulder blades toward your inner elbows. With an exhalation, lift your rib cage from the bottom tips of your shoulder blades and extend your arms.

In Urdhva Dhanurasana, draw the top edges of your shoulder blades away from your upper back, and lift the bottom tips of your shoulder blades toward your kidneys. At the same time, lengthen your outer armpits and lift the sides of your chest. To move deeper into the pose, lift the inner corners of your shoulder blades away from your neck, lengthen from the outer corners of your shoulder blades down through your arms, and let the bottom tips of your shoulder blades move laterally away from your spine. In Urdhva Dhanurasana, the traffic circle of the shoulder blades moves in reverse.

6.15
Urdhva Dhanurasana

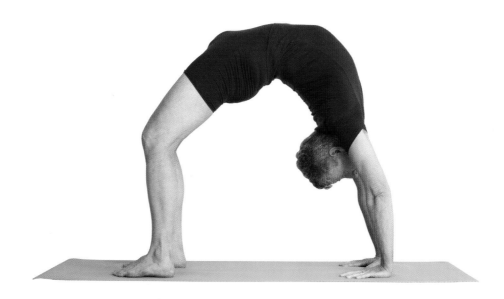

Remain in Urdhva Dhanurasana for 30 seconds. With an inhalation, relax your shoulder blades so that the inner edges and outer edges rest evenly on your rib cage. With an exhalation, lengthen your outer armpits, turn the outer edges of your shoulder blades to face your rib cage, and lengthen the sides of your chest. Balance your rib cage evenly between the outer edges of your shoulder blades.

To come out of the pose, keep your shoulder blades in firm contact with your rib cage as you lower yourself to the floor. Then bring your arms down by your sides, and rest in this position until your breath returns to normal. Repeat Urdhva Dhanurasana two to six times.

RELATED POSE. Viparita Dandasana

6.16
Bharadvajasana II

BHARADVAJASANA II
SIMPLE SEATED TWIST II

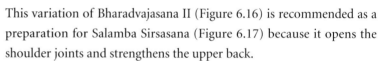

PROPS
- 1 nonskid mat
- 1 blanket

OPTIONAL PROPS
- 1 block or blanket
- 1 strap

This variation of Bharadvajasana II (Figure 6.16) is recommended as a preparation for Salamba Sirsasana (Figure 6.17) because it opens the shoulder joints and strengthens the upper back.

Sit on a folded blanket with your legs extended. Bend your right leg into Virasana (Hero Pose, Figure 5.24), with the top of your right foot on the floor beside your outer right hip. Bring your left leg into Padmasana (Lotus Pose, Figure 3.21), with your left foot resting on your right thigh. (If you have knee problems or tightness in your hip joints, place your left foot on the floor near your inner right thigh. Use a block or blanket to support your left knee, if your knee does not touch the floor.)

Bend your elbows and place your fingertips on the floor close to your outer hips. With an inhalation, widen the top edges of your shoulder blades away from your spine, and lift the inner edges of your shoulder blades away from your kidneys. You can let your head drop back, but only if it feels comfortable on your neck. With an exhalation, keep your left shoulder blade flat against your rib cage as you bring your left forearm behind your back and take hold of your left foot. (If you are unable

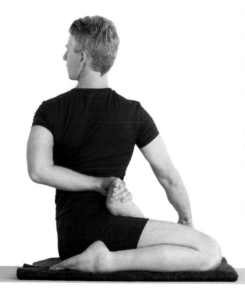

to reach your foot, hold with a strap around your left ankle.) Then lift your head and turn to look over your left shoulder. Press your right hand on your outer left thigh with your arm fully extended.

In Bharadvajasana II, firm the outer edge of your left shoulder blade as you draw the bottom tip of the shoulder blade toward your spine. Bring the inner edge of your left shoulder blade flatter against your back rib cage, and move the top edge of your left shoulder blade away from your spine. Then move the bottom tip of your right shoulder blade laterally away from your spine, and turn from the outer edge of your right shoulder blade.

Maintain this position for 1 minute. With an inhalation, soften the muscles that grip the surface of your left shoulder blade. With an exhalation, move the bottom tip of your left shoulder blade toward your spine and the bottom tip of your right shoulder blade away from your spine. Encourage the circular movement of your shoulder blades with a minimum of effort. When you feel ready, repeat to the other side.

6.17
Salamba Sirsasana

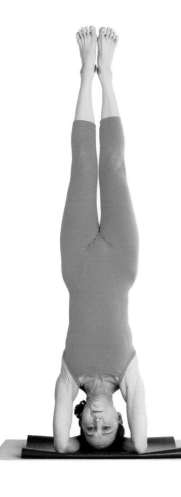

SALAMBA SIRSASANA
HEADSTAND

PROPS

• set up as determined in Chapter 2

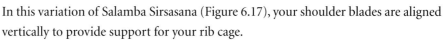

In this variation of Salamba Sirsasana (Figure 6.17), your shoulder blades are aligned vertically to provide support for your rib cage.

Come into Salamba Sirsasana as described in Chapter 2. Widen your collarbones and lift the sides of your chest away from your inner elbows. Let your rib cage rest back against your shoulder blades, and release your shoulder blades away from your spine. If your floating ribs protrude, press the top edges of your shoulder blades against your upper back, and lift the bottom tips away from your elbows to align your shoulder blades vertically. Then lengthen the back of your arms from the outer corners of your shoulder blades, and lift the inner corners of your shoulder blades away from your neck.

Remain in Salamba Sirsasana for 3 to 5 minutes. Lift the bottom tips of your shoulder blades away from your elbows, and firm the outer edges of your shoulder blades against the sides of your rib cage. Balance your weight evenly between your outer shoulder blades. To come out of the pose, stabilize your shoulder blades, release your inner groins, and lower your legs. Rest in Adho Mukha Virasana (Child's Pose, Figure 3.11b).

SALAMBA SARVANGASANA
SHOULDERSTAND

PROPS
• set up as determined in Chapter 1

In this variation of Salamba Sarvangasana (Figure 6.18), the movement of the shoulder blades helps to free the back rib cage, open the shoulders, and protect the neck.

Come into Salamba Sarvangasana as described in Chapter 1. Widen your shoulders, lengthen the back of your arms toward your elbows, and release the top edges of your shoulder blades away from your upper back. At the same time, soften the eyes of your chest, and lift the bottom tips of your shoulder blades away from your elbows. Repeat these adjustments two or three times until your shoulder blades are vertically aligned.

Then observe the top edges of your shoulder blades. If the inner corners of your shoulder blades press into your blanket more heavily than the outer corners, the weight of your body is falling on your neck, rather than on your arms and shoulders. To adjust your shoulder blades, lift the inner corners away from the base of your neck, and press the outer corners down toward your shoulders. At the same time, move the bottom tips of your shoulder blades laterally away from your spine, and lift the back of your rib cage. Repeat this adjustment two or three times so that you feel less weight on your neck and more weight on your arms and outer shoulders.

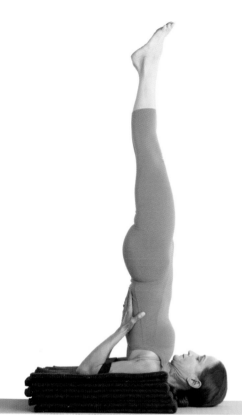

6.18
Salamba Sarvangasana

Finally, bring your awareness to the gap between the outer edges of your shoulder blades and the sides of your chest. Widen your midsternum, firm your back armpits, and bring the outer edges of your shoulder blades into firm contact with the sides of your rib cage. Hold this position for 3 to 5 minutes, maintaining the lift and alignment of your shoulder blades. Then, with an exhalation, release your inner groins and lower your legs into Halasana (Figure 6.19a).

RELATED POSE. Setu Bandhasana

HALASANA
PLOUGH POSE

PROPS

• set up as determined in Chapter 1

This variation of Halasana is divided into two phases: an active phase (Figure 6.19a) with your hands supporting your upper back; and a restorative, or restful, phase (Figure 6.19b) with your arms extended overhead.

Come into Halasana from Salamba Sarvangasana as described for Figure 6.18.

Phase 1. Place your hands flat on your back with your fingers pointing toward your waist. Widen your shoulders, lengthen the back of your arms toward your elbows, and lift your shoulder blades away from the floor. Then soften the eyes of your chest, and let the top edges of your shoulder blades release away from the back of your rib cage.

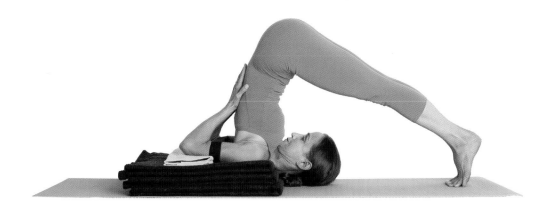

6.19a
Halasana, Phase 1

6.19b
Halasana, Phase 2

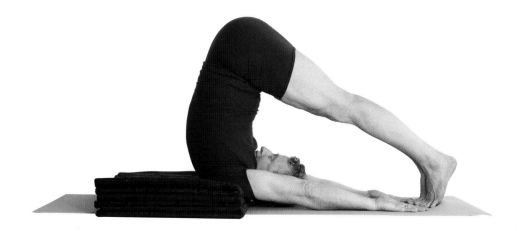

At the same time, lift your kidneys away from your hands, and move your groins away from your kidneys. Remain in this position for 1 more minute.

Phase 2. Now bring your arms to the floor overhead, and lengthen your arms toward your feet. Rest the weight of your body against the top edges of your shoulder blades, and release the bottom tips of your shoulder blades away from your rib cage. Relax your upper back and lift your inner groins away from your kidneys. Remain in this position quietly for 1 more minute.

To come out of the pose, press the back of your hands into the floor, lengthen your arms from the bottom tips of your shoulder blades, and slowly roll down.

JANU SIRSASANA WITH HANDS ON BLOCKS
HEAD-OF-THE-KNEE POSE

PROPS
- 1 nonskid mat
- 2 blocks
- 1 blanket or wedge

OPTIONAL PROP
- 1 block or blanket

6.20a

Janu Sirsasana with Hands on Blocks, Phase 1

This variation of Janu Sirsasana with Hands on Blocks has two phases: a backbend phase, to lengthen your spine and strengthen your upper back (Figure 6.20a), followed by a forward bend phase, to release your spine and broaden your upper back (Figure 6.20b).

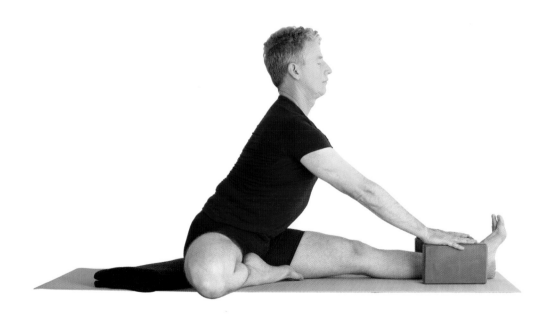

Place a folded blanket or wedge on your nonskid mat. Then sit with your sitting bones on the edge of the blanket or wedge and your legs extended. Bend your right leg and bring your right heel near your right groin with your knee out to the side. (If your right knee does not contact the floor, use a block or blanket to support the knee.)

Phase 1. Place a block on either side of your left foot. (If you are flexible, lay the blocks flat. If you have tight hamstrings, stand the blocks on end.) Then press your fingertips on the floor by your outer hips, and lift the inner edges of your shoulder blades away from your kidneys. Draw your left groin back into your body, and turn your midsternum to face your left leg. With an inhalation, raise your arms overhead and lift from the bottom tips of your shoulder blades. With an exhalation, keep your shoulder blades in firm contact with the back of your upper back, and extend your

6.20b
Janu Sirsasana with Hands on Blocks, Phase 2

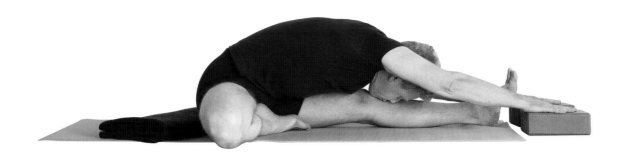

torso over your left leg. Place your hands on the blocks with your palms flat and your arms fully extended.

Maintain this position for several breaths. To bring your rib cage directly over your left leg, move the bottom tip of your right shoulder blade toward the spine and the bottom tip of your left shoulder blade away from the spine.

Phase 2. To move into the forward bend phase of Janu Sirsasana with Hands on Blocks, first, inhale and lift the inner edges of your shoulder blades away from your kidneys to lengthen your upper spine. Then, on an exhalation, slide your blocks forward with your arms fully extended, and lower your chin toward your sternal notch. To release your upper back and deepen your forward bend, let the bottom tips of your shoulder blades move away from your spine, and press the outer edges of your shoulder blades against your rib cage.

To come out of the pose, inhale as you extend your arms and lift up from the bottom tips of your shoulder blades. Then exhale as you lower your arms. Repeat to the other side.

RELATED POSES. Paschimottanasana, other sitting forward bends

UJJAYI PRANAYAMA LYING WITH SHOULDER BLADES SUPPORTED
BASIC YOGA BREATHING

PROPS
- 1 nonskid mat
- 2 blankets
- 1 wedge

This variation of Ujjayi Pranayama Lying with Shoulder Blades Supported (Figure 6.21) releases tension in the shoulder blades and opens the upper lungs.

Fold one blanket in half lengthwise, and place it on your mat to support your rib cage. (When folded, this blanket should measure about 8 inches wide and 30 inches long.) Fold a second blanket in half or in thirds crosswise, and place it at the far end of your first blanket to support your neck and head. Finally, place a wedge in front of your second blanket with the thick edge nearest to the blanket to support your shoulder blades.

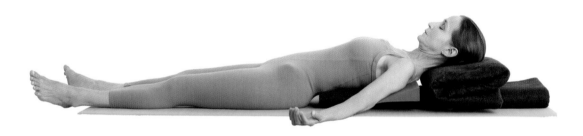

6.21

Ujjayi Pranayama Lying with Shoulder Blades Supported

Lie on your back with your pelvis on the floor and your upper body supported by the blankets. Adjust the height and placement of your props, as necessary. Check that the first blanket supports your lower rib cage, but not your pelvis, and that the second blanket supports the base of your skull and your neck, with your chin slightly tucked. Adjust your shoulder blades so that they rest comfortably on the wedge with the high edge under your shoulders and the thin edge pointing down toward your waist. Lie quietly for several breaths, releasing the weight of your arms and legs with each exhalation.

Begin with a deep, soft exhalation. With a deep, soft inhalation, direct your incoming breath toward your kidneys, and let the top edges of your shoulder blades broaden against the wedge. At the same time, release your collarbones away from your sternal notch, and soften the root of your tongue. With an exhalation, firm the outer edges of your shoulder blades, and let your breath release from the center of your kidneys.

Repeat this cycle for 3 to 4 minutes. Let your shoulder blades soften and broaden with each inhalation, and maintain the position with each exhalation as effortlessly as possible. When you are finished, rest quietly in this position for 1 to 2 minutes; then turn onto your side and sit up.

UJJAYI PRANAYAMA SITTING
BASIC YOGA BREATHING

PROPS	OPTIONAL PROPS
• 1 nonskid mat	• 1 or 2 blocks or blankets
• 1 blanket	• 1 wedge

6.22
Sukhasana

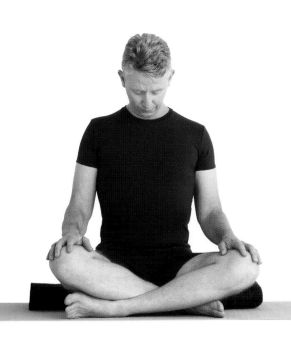

In this variation of Ujjayi Pranayama Sitting, the circular movement of the shoulder blades strengthens the upper back and deepens the breath.

Sit at the edge of a folded blanket in your most comfortable sitting position: Padmasana (Lotus Pose, Figure 3.21), Siddhasana (Perfect Pose, Figure 4.23), Sukhasana (Easy Pose, Figure 6.22), or Virasana (Hero Pose, Figure 5.24). If your knees are not in contact with the floor, use blocks or blankets to support them. (You can also use a wedge under your sitting bones to give an additional lift to your pelvis and spine.)

Bring your elbows to the sides of your waist, so that the backs of your arms are in line with your upper back; then rest the palms of your hands on your thighs. Gently firm your back armpits, and press the outer edges of your shoulder blades evenly on your right and left sides. At the same time, widen your collarbones away from your sternal notch, and drop your chin toward your upper sternum. Close your eyes and draw your eyes deep into their sockets.

Begin with a deep, soft exhalation. With each inhalation, lift the inner edges of your shoulder blades away from your kidneys, release the top edges of your shoulder blades away from your spine, and firm the outer edges of your shoulder blades against the sides of your rib cage. With each exhalation, stabilize your shoulder blades and release your breath from the center of your kidneys. Repeat this cycle for 3 to 5 minutes, integrating the movement of your shoulder blades with the natural rhythm of your breath. Then let your breath return to normal, raise your head, and change the cross of your legs. Repeat for another 3 to 5 minutes; then rest in Savasana (Figure 6.23).

SAVASANA
RELAXATION POSE

PROP
• 1 nonskid mat

OPTIONAL PROP
• 1 blanket

In this variation of Savasana (Figure 6.23), the bottom tips of your shoulder blades move away from the spine to widen your upper back, and the inner corners of your shoulder blades move away from your shoulders to release the base of your neck.

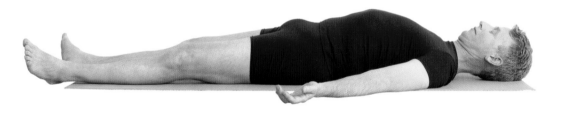

6.23
Savasana

Lie on your back with your knees bent and your feet flat on the floor. (Use a folded blanket under your head and neck if it feels more comfortable.) Place your left hand on your right shoulder, and use your right hand to adjust your left shoulder blade. Move the bottom tip of your shoulder blade away from your spine, and draw the inner corner of your shoulder blade away from the base of your neck. Place your right hand on your left shoulder, and use your left hand to adjust your right shoulder blade in the same way. Then rest your arms on the floor with your palms facing up, without disturbing your shoulder blades. Extend your legs, one at a time; then relax the weight of your legs.

Close your eyes and lengthen from the base of your skull to the crown of your head. Soften the skin of your face, and let your eyes sink deeper into their sockets. Then align yourself with the rhythm of your breath. With an inhalation, release the inner edges of your shoulder blades away from your spine and widen your upper back. With an exhalation, send your breath out from the center of your kidneys. Remain in this position for 5 to 10 minutes. Then bend your knees and turn onto your side before coming up.

▶ PRACTICE SEQUENCE

TADASANA

ADHO MUKHA SVANASANA

UTTHITA TRIKONASANA

UTTANASANA

VIRABHADRASANA I

PADANGUSTHASANA

PARIVRTTA TRIKONASANA

PINCHA MAYURASANA AT THE WALL

USTRASANA

URDHVA HASTASANA II

URDHVA DHANURASANA

BHARADVAJASANA II

SALAMBA SIRSASANA

SALAMBA SARVANGASANA

HALASANA

JANU SIRSASANA WITH HANDS ON BLOCKS

UJJAYI PRANAYAMA LYING WITH SHOULDER BLADES SUPPORTED

UJJAYI PRANAYAMA SITTING

SAVASANA

7 STABILIZE YOUR ELBOWS

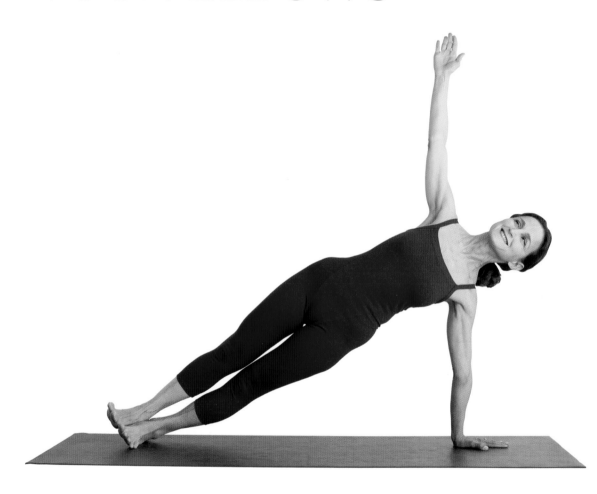

THE PRACTICE SEQUENCE in this chapter focuses on stabilizing your elbow joints in order to strengthen your arms and open your shoulder joints. This sequence is designed especially for those who have a pronounced carrying angle in the arms, who hyperextend their elbow joints, or who complain of weakness in their arms; but the principles presented here for aligning and balancing the arms should benefit all practitioners.

The strength of the arms in arm-balancing poses, such as Adho Mukha Vrksasana at the Wall (Figure 7.16), depends not only on the stability of the elbow joints, but on the shape of the arms themselves. If you have a pronounced carrying angle between your upper arms and forearms, your arms do not provide you with a sturdy vertical support. In my experience, women tend to have a greater carrying angle than men.

To check for a carrying angle, stand in Tadasana (Figure 7.5) with your arms extended forward, and your hands raised to hip level and with your palms turned up. If the bones of your upper arms and fore-arms form a continuous straight line, you do not have a carrying angle. If the line of the forearm bones diverges away from the line of the upper arm bones, the angle of divergence is your carrying angle (Figure 7.1).

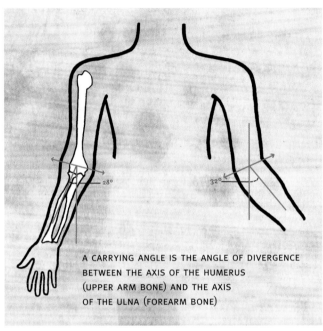

A CARRYING ANGLE IS THE ANGLE OF DIVERGENCE BETWEEN THE AXIS OF THE HUMERUS (UPPER ARM BONE) AND THE AXIS OF THE ULNA (FOREARM BONE)

7.1
Carrying Angle

To estimate the degree of your carrying angle, hold a wedge or other straight edge against your upper inner arm, with your arm extended and your palm turned up. Then calculate the degree of the angle between the wedge and your forearm. If the angle is less than 20 degrees, your arm-balancing poses may not be adversely affected. If the angle is greater than 30 degrees, arm balances will present a definite challenge.

When you calculate your carrying angle, be sure to check both arms. You may find that the carrying angle of one arm is noticeably different from the other. Your right arm and left arm may have very different shapes. A difference in the carrying angle of the two arms is often the root cause of a shoulder imbalance in Adho Mukha Svanasana (Figure 7.14), Adho Mukha Vrksasana at the Wall, and Urdhva Dhanurasana (Figure 3.13).

Observing students who have a pronounced carrying angle, I have noticed how their elbow joints are wide and flat, and relatively unstable. These students tend to hyperextend their elbows, pushing from the point of the elbow toward the elbow crease, which further flattens and destabilizes the joint. For these students, the adjustment frequently recommended by yoga teachers, "Lock your elbows," can be detrimental. Locking the elbows forces the joint open, but weakens the muscles that hold the joint in place.

Instead of locking or pushing into the elbow joint, I prefer to balance and strengthen the muscles around the joint. Stability of the elbow joint comes from narrowing the elbow joint and making it more tubular, not from broadening and flattening it. Narrowing the elbow joint channels the energy through the arm; widening the elbow joint disperses the energy of the arms.

Narrowing and stabilizing your elbow joint involves working from the sides of the joint (the inner and outer elbow), rather than the center (the tip, or point, of the elbow). To clarify what I mean by inner and outer elbows, stand in Tadasana with your arms extended forward and your hands raised to hip level, and with your palms turned up (Figure 7.2). Your inner elbow is the side nearer your rib cage, and your outer elbow is the side farther away. Likewise, your inner wrist is the side of the wrist nearer to your thumb, and your outer wrist is the side nearer to your little finger.

Stabilizing the elbow involves rotating the upper arm and forearm in opposite directions to achieve a dynamic balance. Try this exercise. Stand in Tadasana with your arms extended by your sides. As you firm your inner elbows and lift the sides of your chest, feel how your upper arms roll out. Then lengthen from your outer elbows to your inner wrists, and observe how your forearms roll in. This counterrotation of the forearm and upper arm strengthens your forearms, firms and gently squeezes your elbow joints, and allows your shoulders to open (Figure 7.3).

The strength of your upper arms depends on the balance between your inner and outer triceps (the muscles at the back of your upper arm). The lateral head of your outer triceps originates on your outer arm bone (humerus), close to your outer shoulder. The long head of your inner triceps originates at the outer edge of your shoulder blade and forms the ridge of your outer armpit. (When I ask you later in this chapter

left:
7.2
Inner and Outer Elbows

right:
7.3
*Counterrotation of
Forearms and Upper Arms*

facing page top:
7.4
Inner and Outer Triceps

facing page bottom:
7.5
Tadasana

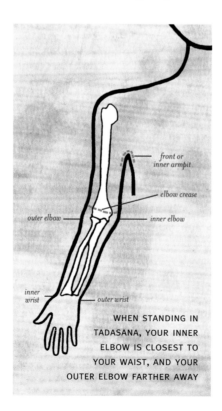

WHEN STANDING IN TADASANA, YOUR INNER ELBOW IS CLOSEST TO YOUR WAIST, AND YOUR OUTER ELBOW FARTHER AWAY

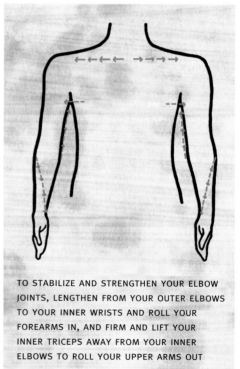

TO STABILIZE AND STRENGTHEN YOUR ELBOW JOINTS, LENGTHEN FROM YOUR OUTER ELBOWS TO YOUR INNER WRISTS AND ROLL YOUR FOREARMS IN, AND FIRM AND LIFT YOUR INNER TRICEPS AWAY FROM YOUR INNER ELBOWS TO ROLL YOUR UPPER ARMS OUT

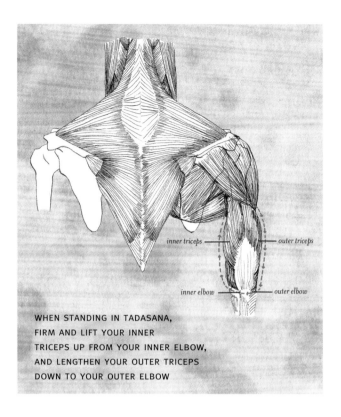

WHEN STANDING IN TADASANA,
FIRM AND LIFT YOUR INNER
TRICEPS UP FROM YOUR INNER ELBOW,
AND LENGTHEN YOUR OUTER TRICEPS
DOWN TO YOUR OUTER ELBOW

to lengthen from your inner elbow to your outer armpit, you are, in fact, activating the whole length of your inner triceps.)

For most people, the outer triceps are tighter and shorter than the inner triceps, and draw up toward the shoulders. The inner triceps tend to be loose and slack, and drop toward the inner elbows. To balance your inner and outer triceps, stand in Tadasana with your arms extended and your elbows at the sides of your waist. Lengthen your outer triceps from your outer shoulders down to your outer elbows, and feel how the ridge of your shoulders softens and widens. At the same time, firm your inner triceps, just above your inner elbows, and draw your inner arms upward. Feel how your chest expands (Figure 7.4).

By stabilizing your elbow joints, the following practice sequence strengthens your arms and upper back, relaxes and broadens your shoulders, and improves the alignment of your whole upper body.

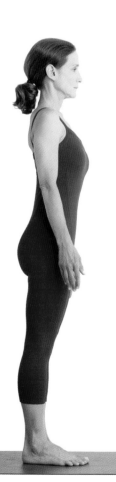

TADASANA
MOUNTAIN POSE

PROP
• 1 nonskid mat

This variation of Tadasana (Figure 7.5) balances the inner and outer triceps to strengthen the arms and open the shoulder joints.

Stand on your mat in Tadasana with your feet together and your arms extended by your sides. Bring your inner elbows in line with the sides of your waist, and turn your palms to face your body. (If you have a carrying angle, your hands may come forward of your legs.) Then adjust your pelvis so that your inner groins are in line with your kidneys, and lift your kidneys away from your inner groins.

In Tadasana, release your collarbones away from your sternal notch and broaden your inner armpits. Lengthen from your inner elbows to your outer armpits to firm your inner triceps and roll your upper arms out. At the same time, lengthen from your outer elbows to your inner wrists to roll your forearms in. Then broaden your palms and gently squeeze your elbow joints—as though you were squeezing an orange.

Maintain this position for 30 seconds. Lengthen your outer triceps from your outer shoulders down to your outer elbows. Firm and lift your inner triceps from your inner elbows to your outer armpits. In particular, firm your inner triceps just above your inner elbows, where they are weakest. Return to Tadasana after every standing pose to center your energy and balance your inner and outer arms.

Practice Notes. If you have a carrying angle, be sure to align your elbows with the sides of your waist when you stand in Tadasana. If you place your hands by your outer legs, your elbows may fall behind your waist; in this case, you will tend to overarch your back and overwork your spine.

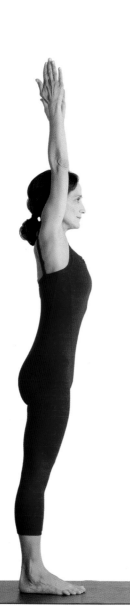

7.6
Urdhva Hastasana I

URDHVA HASTASANA I
MOUNTAIN POSE WITH ARMS OVERHEAD

PROP
• 1 nonskid mat

This variation of Urdhva Hastasana I (Figure 7.6) focuses on the proper alignment of your upper arms when raising your arms overhead.

Stand on your mat in Tadasana (Figure 7.5) with your feet together and your arms by your sides. Adjust your pelvis so that your inner groins are in line with your kidneys, and lift your kidneys away from your inner groins. Release your collarbones away from your sternal notch and broaden your inner armpits. With an inhalation, turn your palms and forearms out. With an exhalation, keep your elbows in line with the sides of your waist as you raise your arms out to the side and overhead.

In Urdhva Hastasana I, press your outer triceps toward each other, and lengthen from your outer armpits to your inner elbows evenly on both sides. Then gently squeeze your elbow joints, and lengthen from your outer elbows to your inner wrists. Let your elbow creases face the mounds of your thumbs.

Maintain this position for 30 seconds. Check that your elbow joints are directly in line with the sides of your waist, neither too far forward nor too far back. When your elbows are in line with the sides of your waist, your upper arms can lift vertically, creating maximum space in your shoulder joints.

To come out of the pose, inhale and turn your palms out; then exhale and keep your elbows in line with the sides of your waist as you lower your arms.

Practice Notes. If you have a pronounced carrying angle, you may have difficulty aligning your arms when you bring them overhead. If your forearms are vertical, your upper arms will be forward of the sides of your rib cage, and your shoulder joints will not be fully open. To align your upper arms vertically and open your shoulder joints, keep your elbows in line with the sides of your waist as you raise your arms overhead.

RELATED POSE. Virabhadrasana I

7.7
*Ardha Uttanasana
with Hands on the Wall*

ARDHA UTTANASANA WITH HANDS ON THE WALL
RIGHT ANGLE POSE

PROPS
- 1 nonskid mat
- 1 wall

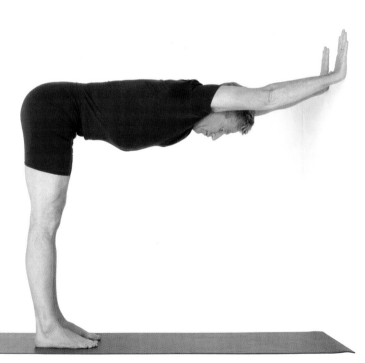

In this variation of Ardha Uttanasana with Hands on the Wall (Figure 7.7), your upper arms are the key to proper alignment of your upper body.

Stand on your mat in Tadasana (Figure 7.5) facing a wall, a forearm's distance away from the wall. Press your elbows against the sides of your waist, and place your hands on the wall with your palms flat and your fingers pointing upward. Then step your feet back until your arms are fully extended and your heels are in line with your sitting bones. Check that your upper arms, not your forearms, are parallel to the floor.

In Ardha Uttanasana with Hands on the Wall, broaden your palms against the wall, and draw your inner groins away from your kidneys to lengthen your spine. Turn your elbow creases to face the mounds of your thumbs, and lengthen your forearms from your outer elbows to your inner wrists, pressing the bottom knuckles of your index fingers into the wall. At the same time, stabilize your elbow joints and lengthen your outer armpits away from your inner elbows.

Maintain this position for several breaths. Lengthen your outer triceps from your outer shoulders toward your outer elbows, and firm your inner triceps just above your inner elbows to make contact with the bone. If your outer triceps are tight, soften and lengthen them. If your outer triceps are weak, firm and lengthen them. If your outer triceps are in between, simply lengthen them.

To come out of the pose, inhale as you lift your head and shoulders, and exhale as you step forward into Tadasana.

Practice Notes. If you have a pronounced carrying angle, you may need to place your hands higher on the wall, so that your upper arms are parallel to the floor. If you place your hands at hip level, your upper arms and shoulder girdle will sink lower than your pelvis, and you will lose the extension of your spine.

ADHO MUKHA SVANASANA WITH HANDS ON BLOCKS
DOWNWARD-FACING DOG POSE VARIATION

PROPS
- 1 nonskid mat
- 2 blocks
- 1 wall

7.8
Adho Mukha Svanasana with Hands on Blocks

This variation of Adho Mukha Svanasana with Hands on Blocks (Figure 7.8) is recommended for those with a pronounced carrying angle, and is helpful for anyone with tight shoulders.

Place two blocks lengthwise and shoulder-width apart against the base of a wall; put a nonskid mat under the blocks to prevent them from slipping. Start in a kneeling position with your palms flat on the blocks, your hip joints directly over your

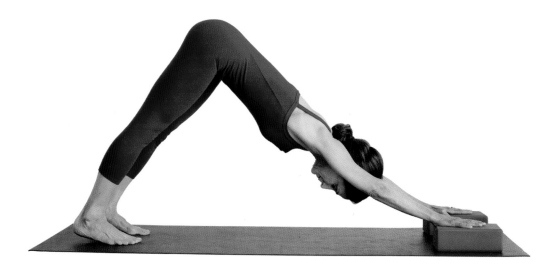

knees, and your toes turned under. Press the bottom knuckles of your index fingers into the blocks, and turn your elbow creases to face the mounds of your thumbs. With an inhalation, lengthen down from your outer elbows to your inner wrists, and lift up from your inner elbows. With an exhalation, keep your elbow joints firm as you lift your pelvis and straighten your legs.

In Adho Mukha Svanasana with Hands on Blocks, lift your inner groins away from your kidneys, and lengthen the sides of your chest. Press the bottom knuckles of your index fingers into the blocks, and lengthen your forearms from your outer elbows to your inner wrists. At the same time, firm your inner triceps just above your inner elbows and lengthen your outer armpits evenly on your right and left sides. Repeat these instructions two or three times.

Maintain this position for 1 to 2 minutes. Lengthen from your outer shoulders to your outer elbows so that your outer triceps make contact with your outer arm bones. Lengthen your outer armpits away from your inner elbows, and firm your inner triceps against your inner arm bones. Relax your shoulders, but keep your elbows stable.

To come out of the pose, bend your knees and rest in Adho Mukha Virasana (Child's Pose, Figure 3.11b) for several breaths.

Practice Notes. If you have a carrying angle, using blocks under your hands in Adho Mukha Svanasana will bring your elbows and shoulders into better alignment. If you have a carrying angle but don't use blocks, your elbows may sink toward the floor and prevent your shoulders from opening. In this case, lift your lower forearms away from your wrist joints to stabilize your elbows and allow your shoulders to release down.

VIRABHADRASANA II
WARRIOR POSE II

PROP
• 1 nonskid mat

This variation of Virabhadrasana II (Figure 7.9) strengthens your upper back and arms by activating your inner and outer triceps.

Stand on your mat in Tadasana (Figure 7.5), and separate your legs about 4½ feet apart. Turn your left foot in 30 degrees and your right foot out 90 degrees. Extend your arms by the sides of your body so that your elbows are in line with your waist; then lengthen your spine. With an inhalation, keep your elbows in line with the sides of your waist as you raise your arms to shoulder height. With an exhalation, bend your right knee to form a right angle, and turn your head to look over your right hand.

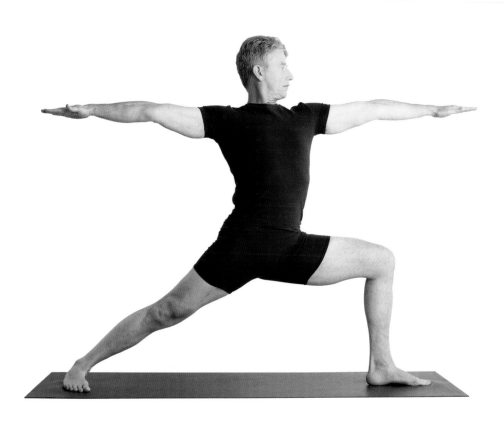

7.9
Virabhadrasana II

In Virabhadrasana II, bring your inner groins in line with your kidneys, and lift your kidneys away from your inner groins. Release your collarbones away from your sternal notch and broaden your front armpits. Then lengthen from the center of your back armpits toward your inner elbows so that your inner triceps press firmly against the bone. Turn your elbow creases to face your thumbs, and lengthen your forearms from your outer elbows to your inner wrists.

Maintain this position for 30 seconds. Turn your head and neck to look over your right hand. If your rib cage turns to the right, lift your right kidney away from your right groin, and lengthen from your outer right armpit to your inner right elbow so that your rib cage faces directly forward. Then gently squeeze your elbow joints and widen your shoulders.

To come out of the pose, inhale as you straighten your right leg, and exhale as you lower your elbows to the sides of your waist. Repeat to the other side.

RELATED POSES. Utthita Trikonasana, Ardha Chandrasana

UTTANASANA WITH HANDS ON A BLOCK
STANDING FORWARD BEND

PROPS

- 1 nonskid mat
- 1 block

This variation of Uttanasana with Hands on a Block (Figure 7.10) aligns the arms, stabilizes the elbow joints, and lengthens the spine.

Place a block on end vertically about 18 inches in front of you. Then stand in Tadasana (Figure 7.5) with your feet a few inches apart and your arms by your sides. With an inhalation, keep your elbows in line with the sides of your waist as you raise your arms out to the side and overhead. With an exhalation, keep your elbow joints firm as you draw your groins into your body and lengthen your torso forward. Place your fingers on top of the block, and press your thumbs into the nearest side of the block. Then straighten your arms, firm your inner elbows, and slide the block forward, if necessary. (If you are very flexible, you can turn the block on its side.)

In Uttanasana with Hands on a Block, lift your groins away from your kidneys, and lengthen your kidneys away from your groins to release your lumbar spine. Lengthen your outer armpits away from your inner elbows to release the sides of your chest. Then lift your inner elbows toward the ceiling, and lengthen from your outer elbows to your inner wrists to release your shoulders. Let your elbow creases face the mounds of your thumbs.

7.10

Uttanasana with Hands on a Block

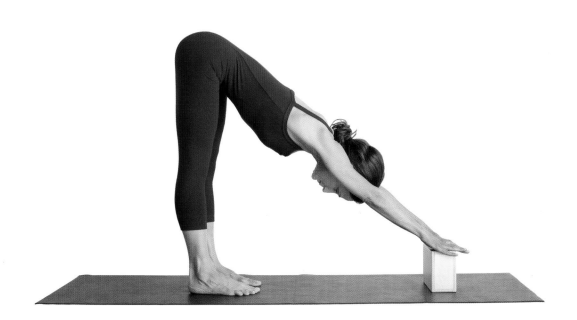

Maintain this position for about 1 minute. Lengthen your outer armpits away from your inner elbows, and firm your inner triceps. At the same time, widen your inner armpits and lengthen your outer triceps toward your outer elbows to open your shoulders.

To come out of the pose, place your hands on your hips and firm your inner elbows. With an inhalation, lift your torso to an upright position. With an exhalation, extend your arms by your sides and return to Tadasana.

RELATED POSES. Practice these poses with your arms extended forward, to align your arms and stabilize your elbows: Prasarita Padottanasana, Parsvottanasana.

UTTHITA PARSVAKONASANA WITH A BLOCK
EXTENDED SIDE-ANGLE POSE

PROPS
- 1 nonskid mat
- 1 block

7.11

Utthita Parsvakonasana with a Block

In Utthita Parsvakonasana with a Block (Figure 7.11), place your palm on a block by your outer ankle to help stabilize your elbow joint and strengthen your arm.

Start in Tadasana (Figure 7.5), and separate your legs about 4½ feet apart. Turn your left foot in 30 degrees and your right foot out 90 degrees. With an inhalation, keep your elbows in line with the sides of your waist as you raise your arms to shoulder height. With an exhalation, bend your right knee to form a square, and extend the right side of your rib cage along your right thigh.

Rest your left arm along the left side of your rib cage so that your left elbow touches the left side of your waist. Keep your left elbow in line with the left side of your waist as you swing your left arm overhead. Place the palm of your right hand on the block by your outer right ankle.

In Utthita Parsvakonasana with a Block, bring your inner groins in line with your kidneys, and lengthen your kidneys away from your inner groins. On your right (bent-leg) side, turn your elbow crease to face the mound of your thumb, and broaden your palm on the block. Lengthen from your outer elbow to your inner wrist, and lift your outer armpit away from your inner elbow. On your left (extended-leg) side, lengthen from your outer armpit to your inner elbow. Then firm your inner elbow, and lengthen from your outer elbow to your inner wrist. Keep your palm broad and your fingers long.

Maintain this position for 30 seconds. Check the alignment of your rib cage. If your rib cage turns toward the floor, broaden your inner right armpit, and lift your rib cage away from your inner right elbow so that the front of your rib cage turns toward the ceiling.

To come out of the pose, lengthen your left arm and swing your left elbow toward the left side of your waist. With an inhalation, straighten your right leg and lift your torso to an upright position. With an exhalation, turn your feet forward; then repeat to the other side.

RELATED POSES. Utthita Trikonasana, Ardha Chandrasana, Parivrtta Ardha Chandrasana, Parivrtta Trikonasana

PADANGUSTHASANA
TOE-HOLDING POSE

7.12
Padangusthasana

PROP	OPTIONAL PROP
• 1 nonskid mat	• 1 block

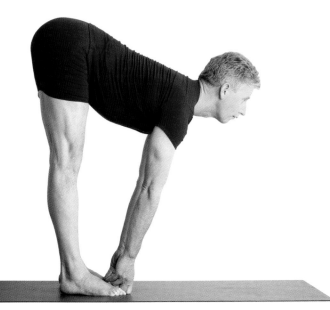

This variation of Padangusthasana (Figure 7.12) strengthens the arms and lengthens the spine.

Stand on your mat in Tadasana (Figure 7.5) with your feet a few inches apart and your arms by your sides. With an inhalation, keep your elbows in line with the sides of your waist as you raise your arms out to the side and overhead. With an exhalation, keep your elbow joints firm as you draw your groins back into your body and lengthen your torso forward. When your spine is parallel to the floor, wrap your second and third fingers around your big toes, and press your thumbs into the floor facing each other. (If you are unable to reach your toes without rounding your back, place a block on end in front of your feet, and rest your hands on the block.)

In Padangusthasana, lengthen your kidneys away from your groins, and lift your groins away from your kidneys. Turn your elbow creases to face the mounds of your thumbs. Then lengthen down from your outer elbows to your inner wrists, and press your thumbs into the floor. At the same time, lift from your inner elbows, and firm your inner triceps into the bone. Maintain this position for several breaths.

To come out of the pose, first, place your hands on your hips. Then lift your torso with an inhalation, and return to Tadasana with an exhalation.

RELATED POSE. Prasarita Padottanasana (Phase 1)

7.13
Virabhadrasana I

VIRABHADRASANA I
WARRIOR POSE I

PROP
• 1 nonskid mat

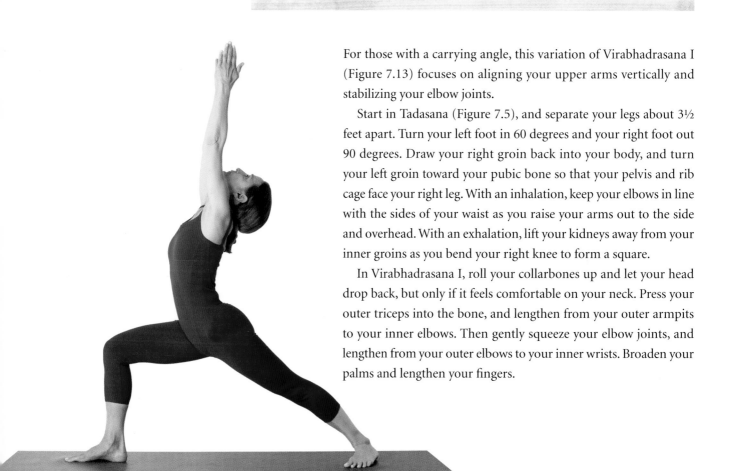

For those with a carrying angle, this variation of Virabhadrasana I (Figure 7.13) focuses on aligning your upper arms vertically and stabilizing your elbow joints.

Start in Tadasana (Figure 7.5), and separate your legs about 3½ feet apart. Turn your left foot in 60 degrees and your right foot out 90 degrees. Draw your right groin back into your body, and turn your left groin toward your pubic bone so that your pelvis and rib cage face your right leg. With an inhalation, keep your elbows in line with the sides of your waist as you raise your arms out to the side and overhead. With an exhalation, lift your kidneys away from your inner groins as you bend your right knee to form a square.

In Virabhadrasana I, roll your collarbones up and let your head drop back, but only if it feels comfortable on your neck. Press your outer triceps into the bone, and lengthen from your outer armpits to your inner elbows. Then gently squeeze your elbow joints, and lengthen from your outer elbows to your inner wrists. Broaden your palms and lengthen your fingers.

Maintain this position for 30 seconds. Widen your groins and lift your kidneys away from your groins. Soften and lengthen your outer triceps from your outer shoulders to your outer elbows. Firm your inner triceps just above your inner elbows to make contact with your inner arm bones. Lift your elbow joints away from the sides of your waist.

To come out of the pose, lift your elbow joints and straighten your right leg with an inhalation. With an exhalation, keep your elbows in line with the sides of your waist as you lower your arms. Then repeat to the other side.

ADHO MUKHA SVANASANA
DOWNWARD-FACING DOG POSE

PROP
• 1 nonskid mat

7.14
Adho Mukha Svanasana

If you have a carrying angle, come into this variation of Adho Mukha Svanasana (Figure 7.14) with your upper back rounded to avoid dropping your elbows.

Start on your nonskid mat in a kneeling position with the mounds of your thumbs in line with the center of your shoulder joints and with your feet and knees in line with the center of your hip joints. Turn your elbow creases to face the mound of your thumbs and broaden your palms. With an inhalation, lengthen down from your outer elbows to your inner wrists, lift away from your inner elbows, and let your upper back round toward the ceiling. With an exhalation, keep your elbow joints firm as you lift your pelvis and straighten your legs.

In Adho Mukha Svanasana, lift your inner groins away from your kidneys and lengthen the sides of your chest. Press the bottom knuckles of your index fingers into the floor, and lengthen your forearms from your outer elbows to your inner wrists. At the same time, firm your inner triceps and lengthen your outer armpits away from your inner elbows.

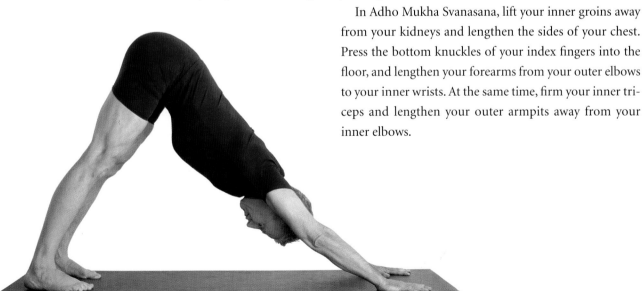

Maintain this position for 1 to 2 minutes. Relax your shoulders and stabilize your elbow joints. Lift your inner triceps away from your inner elbows, and lengthen your outer triceps down to your outer elbows. If your outer triceps are tight, soften and lengthen your outer triceps. If your outer triceps are lax, firm and lengthen your outer triceps.

To come out of the pose, bend your knees and rest your torso on your thighs in Adho Mukha Virasana (Child's Pose, Figure 3.11b) for several breaths.

Practice Notes. Students often ask in Adho Mukha Svanasana, "Which way should my elbow creases face? Should they face each other or face toward the ceiling?" My answer is, "Somewhere in between."

If your elbow creases face toward the ceiling in Adho Mukha Svanasana, you are probably hyperextending your elbows and rolling your forearms out. In this case, turn your elbow creases to face the mounds of your thumbs, and lengthen from your outer elbows to your inner wrists to roll your forearms in.

If your elbow creases face each other or toward the floor, you are probably gripping your shoulders and rolling your upper arms in. In this case, turn your elbow creases to face your thumbs, and firm your inner triceps just above your inner elbows so that your upper arms turn out. When your arms are properly balanced, your forearms roll in and your upper arms roll out. This counteraction firms and stabilizes your elbow joints.

VASISTHASANA
SIDE PLANK POSE

PROP
• 1 nonskid mat

OPTIONAL PROP
• 1 wall

This variation of Vasisthasana (Figure 7.15a) strengthens your arms and improves your balance by stabilizing your elbow joints.

Start in Adho Mukha Svanasana as described for Figure 7.14. With an inhalation, lift your inner groins away from your kidneys, and lengthen the sides of your chest away from your inner elbows. With an exhalation, swing your torso forward into a plank position so that your shoulders are directly over your hands. (If you are a beginning student or have a shoulder injury, hold this position for 30 seconds, and then return to Adho Mukha Svanasana.)

To come into Vasisthasana, turn your right elbow crease to face the mound of your right thumb, and lengthen from your outer right elbow to your inner wrist. At the same time, firm and lift your inner triceps away from your inner right elbow. With an inhalation, place your left foot against your right foot, and turn onto the outer edge of your right foot. With an exhalation, shift the weight of your body onto your right hand, and raise your left arm toward the ceiling.

In Vasisthasana, check that your right shoulder is directly over your right hand, so that your right forearm is vertically aligned. Turn your right elbow crease to face the mound of your right thumb. Then lengthen down from your outer right elbow to your inner right wrist, and lift your rib cage away from your inner right elbow. Check that your left elbow is directly over your left shoulder, so that your upper left arm is vertically aligned. Turn your left elbow crease to face the mound of your left thumb. Then lengthen from your outer left armpit to your inner left elbow, and lift your left forearm from your outer left elbow to your inner left wrist. Broaden the palm of your left hand and lengthen your fingers.

Maintain this position for 30 seconds. Broaden your inner right armpit, and lengthen your outer triceps from your outer right shoulder to your outer right elbow. At the same time, firm your inner right triceps and lift your outer right armpit away from your inner right elbow. Let your rib cage lift and turn away from the outer edge of your right shoulder blade. Then bring the sides of your waist in line with your elbows to adjust your pelvis. If your balance is steady, turn your head toward the ceiling.

To come out of the pose, bring your left hand back to the floor, return to Adho Mukha Svanasana, and repeat to the other side.

Practice Notes. If balancing in Vasisthasana is difficult for you, practice Vasisthasana Facing a Wall (Figure 7.15b). Start in Adho Mukha Svanasana with your left

7.15a
Vasisthasana

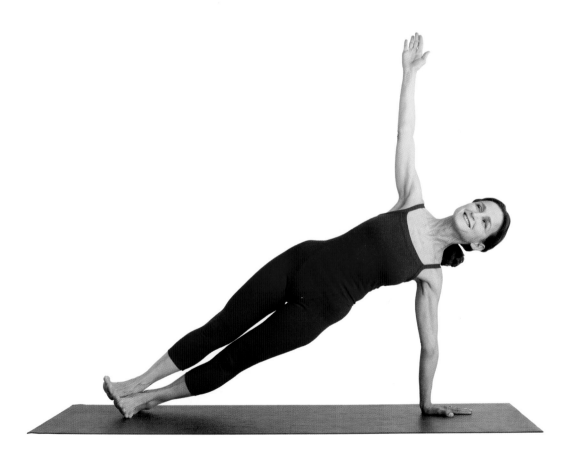

side about 6 inches from the wall. Come into Vasisthasana with your right arm as the supporting arm, so that the front of your body is facing the wall. Place your left hand on the wall to give you support, and work with your right arm and rib cage as previously described. Then repeat to the other side.

RELATED POSE. Ardha Chandrasana

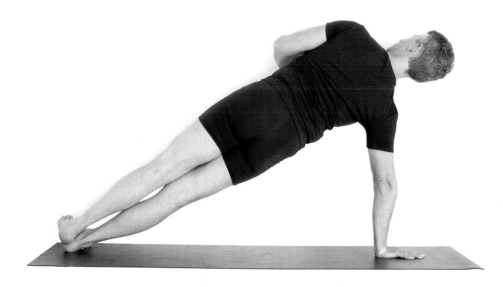

right:
7.15b
Vasisthasana
Facing a Wall

below:
7.16
Adho Mukha Vrksasana
at the Wall

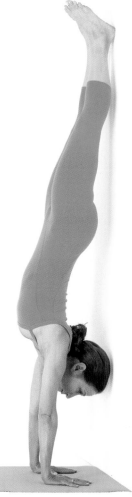

ADHO MUKHA VRKSASANA AT THE WALL
HANDSTAND VARIATION

PROPS
- 1 nonskid mat
- 1 wall

If you have a carrying angle, your forearms—*not* your upper arms—should be vertically aligned in Adho Mukha Vrksasana at the Wall (Figure 7.16).

Start in Adho Mukha Svanasana (Figure 7.14) with your hands about 6 inches from the wall. Turn your elbow creases to face the mounds of your thumbs, and lengthen from your outer elbows to your inner wrists. At the same time, firm your inner triceps just above your inner elbows, and bring your shoulders directly over your hands. With an inhalation, bend one leg and step the foot a few inches closer to the wall. With an exhalation, keep your other leg straight as you swing it in a wide arc toward the wall. Let the momentum of your straight leg draw your bent leg away from the floor. Rest your heels on the wall, but not your pelvis.

In Adho Mukha Vrksasana at the Wall, turn your elbow creases to face the mounds of your thumbs. Lengthen from your outer elbows to your inner wrists, and move your elbows toward the wall to keep your forearms vertically aligned. Lift the sides of your rib cage away from your inner elbows to open your chest. Then lift your inner groins away from your kidneys as you lengthen your legs. When you make these adjustments, you may find that your legs are drawn away from the wall and you are balancing without support. Enjoy the moment!

Maintain this position for 30 seconds. Turn your sternal notch toward the base of your throat, and lift your head from the base of your skull to face the floor. Broaden your inner armpits and lengthen your outer triceps from your outer shoulders to your outer elbows. Firm your inner triceps and lift your outer armpits away from your inner elbows.

When you feel that you are losing the lift of your spine, stay 2 or 3 more seconds and then come down. Rest in Uttanasana (Figure 6.8) until your breathing returns to normal. Repeat Adho Mukha Vrksasana at the Wall two or three times.

Practice Notes. If you have a pronounced carrying angle, you may need to place your hands farther away from the wall. If your hands are too close to the wall, you will not have enough space to align your forearms vertically.

URDHVA MUKHA SVANASANA
UPWARD-FACING DOG POSE

PROPS
- 1 nonskid mat
- 1 blanket

OPTIONAL PROP
- 2 blocks

7.17
Urdhva Mukha Svanasana

This variation of Urdhva Mukha Svanasana (Figure 7.17) stabilizes your elbows and strengthens your arms.

Lie face down on your mat with your pelvis on a folded blanket. Extend your arms by your sides and rest your forehead on the floor. Then bend your elbows and place your hands flat on the floor by the sides of your waist (*not* by the sides of your

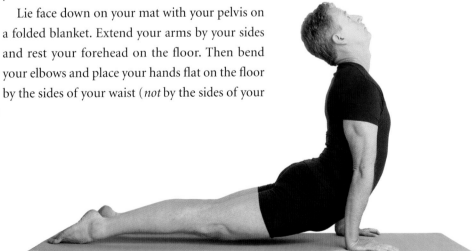

rib cage) so that your upper arms are parallel to each other. With an inhalation, raise your head, release your collarbones away from your sternal notch, and broaden your inner armpits. With an exhalation, keep your inner elbows firm as you lift your rib cage and straighten your arms. (If your arms are short in proportion to the length of your torso, use blocks under your palms to give additional height. If you have wrist problems, use blocks under the heels of your hands to take the pressure off your wrists. In this case, curl your fingers over the front edges of the blocks.)

In Urdhva Mukha Svanasana, lengthen your inner groins away from your kidneys and lift your kidneys away from your inner groins. If you hyperextend your elbows, turn your elbow creases to face the mounds of your thumbs, and lengthen your forearms from your outer elbows to your inner wrists. At the same time, lift your outer armpits away from your inner elbows and firm your inner triceps.

Maintain this position for 30 seconds. Press your outer triceps toward each other, and lengthen from your outer shoulders to your outer elbows. At the same time, firm your inner triceps and lift away from your inner elbow joints.

To come out of the pose, keep your inner elbows firm as you bend your arms and lower your torso to the floor. Repeat this pose two or three times.

RELATED POSES. Salabhasana, Ustrasana

CAUTION

If you are a beginning student or have not attempted this variation before, practice with the wedge at the wall.

As you gain more experience, you can try it away from the wall, as shown in Figure 7.18.

URDHVA DHANURASANA WITH HANDS ON A WEDGE
UPWARD-FACING BOW POSE VARIATION

PROP
- 1 nonskid mat
- 1 wedge

OPTIONAL PROP
- 1 wall
- 1 strap

Urdhva Dhanurasana with Hands on a Wedge (Figure 7.18) takes pressure off your wrists and helps to straighten your arms and open your shoulders.

Place a wedge on a nonskid mat at the base of a wall so that the thick edge of the wedge is against the wall. Then lie on your back with your head near the wall, and place your hands on the wedge. (If you are unable to straighten your arms or if you have a pronounced carrying angle and your arms feel weak, use a strap around your upper arms to stabilize your elbows.)

Bend your knees and place your feet on the floor in line with your sitting bones and about 6 inches away. With an inhalation, lengthen from your outer armpits to your inner elbows, and move the points of your elbows away from the bottom tips of your shoulder blades. With an exhalation, lift the bottom tips of your shoulder blades away from your elbows as you raise your rib cage and straighten your arms.

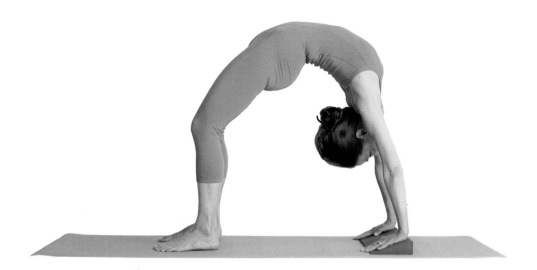

7.18

Urdhva Dhanurasana with Hands on a Wedge

In Urdhva Dhanurasana with Hands on a Wedge, lift your kidneys away from your inner groins, and move your inner groins away from your kidneys to bring your rib cage and pelvis into balance. Walk your feet toward your hands, if necessary. Then turn your elbow creases to face the mounds of your thumbs. Lengthen your forearms from your outer elbows to your inner wrists, and lift the bottom tips of your shoulder blades away from your inner elbows to create space in your shoulder joints.

Maintain this position for 30 seconds. Turn your sternal notch toward the base of your throat, and lift your head from the base of your skull. Broaden your inner armpits and lengthen your outer triceps from your outer shoulders to your outer elbows. At the same time, firm your inner triceps and lift the sides of your rib cage away from your inner elbows. Stabilize your elbow joints and allow your shoulders to open.

To come out of the pose, keep your inner elbows firm as you bend your arms and lower your torso to the floor. Lie on your back until your breath returns to normal. Then repeat three to six times.

BHARADVAJASANA II
SIMPLE SEATED TWIST II

PROPS
- 1 nonskid mat
- 1 blanket

OPTIONAL PROPS
- 1 block or blanket
- 1 strap

This variation of Bharadvajasana II (Figure 7.19) creates space in your shoulder joints by firming the elbow and activating both inner and outer triceps.

Place a folded blanket on your mat, and sit on the blanket with your legs extended.

Bend your right leg into Virasana (Hero Pose, Figure 5.24), with the top of your right foot on the floor beside your outer right hip. Bring your left leg into Padmasana (Lotus Pose, Figure 3.21), with your left foot resting on your right thigh. (If you have knee problems or tightness in your hip joints, place your left foot on the floor near your inner right thigh. Use a block or blanket to support your left knee, if your knee does not touch the floor.)

Bend your elbows and place your fingertips on the floor behind your pelvis. Bring your upper arms parallel to each other, and firm your inner elbows. With an inhalation, broaden your inner armpits, lengthen from your outer armpits to your inner elbows, and lift the sides of your chest. With an exhalation, take hold of your left foot with your left hand, and press your right hand against your outer left knee. (If you are unable to reach your left foot, loop a strap around your left ankle.)

In Bharadvajasana II, lift your kidneys away from your inner groins, and turn your head to look over your left shoulder. With your left arm behind your back, firm your inner left elbow, and lift the left side of your rib cage to open your left shoulder. Lengthen your left forearm from your outer left elbow to your inner left wrist to deepen the twist from the right side of your waist. With your right arm fully extended, turn your right elbow crease to face the mound of your right thumb. Then lengthen from your outer right elbow to your inner right wrist, and firm your inner right elbow to lift your lower abdomen.

Maintain this position for 1 minute. Broaden your inner left armpit, and lengthen your outer left triceps from your outer left shoulder to your outer left elbow. At the same time, firm your inner left triceps against the bone, and lift your outer left armpit away from your inner left elbow. Then gently squeeze both elbow joints, and lift your kidneys away from your inner groins.

7.19
Bharadvajasana II

To come out of the pose, release the hold of your left foot, return to a sitting position with your legs extended, and repeat to the other side.

RELATED POSES. Other sitting twists

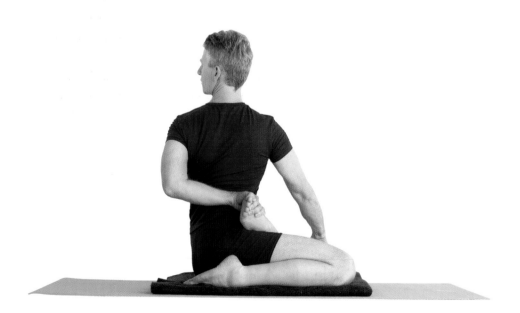

ARDHA SIRSASANA WITH FOREARMS ON THE WALL
HALF HEADSTAND

PROPS
- 1 nonskid mat
- 1 wall

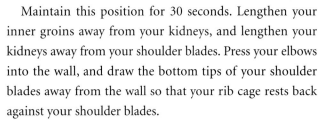

7.20
Ardha Sirsasana with Forearms on the Wall

Ardha Sirsasana with Forearms on the Wall (Figure 7.20) teaches you how to lengthen the sides of your rib cage away from your elbows and balance the weight on your forearms, in preparation for Salamba Sirsasana (Figure 7.21).

Stand on your mat in Tadasana (Figure 7.5) facing a wall approximately 2 feet away. Bend your elbows, interlock your fingers, and place your forearms and outer hands on the wall with your elbows at hip level. Then walk your feet back so that your spine is fully extended and your heels are in line with your sitting bones.

In Ardha Sirsasana with Forearms on the Wall, lengthen your outer hands away from your outer wrists, and press your forearms into the wall. At the same time, broaden your inner armpits and lengthen your outer armpits away from your inner elbows to lengthen the sides of your chest.

Maintain this position for 30 seconds. Lengthen your inner groins away from your kidneys, and lengthen your kidneys away from your shoulder blades. Press your elbows into the wall, and draw the bottom tips of your shoulder blades away from the wall so that your rib cage rests back against your shoulder blades.

To come out of the pose, first release the interlock of your fingers. Then press your hands into the wall, and step forward into Tadasana. Change the interlock of your fingers and repeat the pose.

Practice Notes. If your weight drops onto your elbows in Salamba Sirsasana and your lower ribs protrude, practice lifting the bottom tips of your shoulder blades away from your elbows in Ardha Sirsasana with Forearms on the Wall before doing Salamba Sirsasana. If this movement does not improve your alignment, try using a lift under your elbows in Salamba Sirsasana as described in Chapter 2.

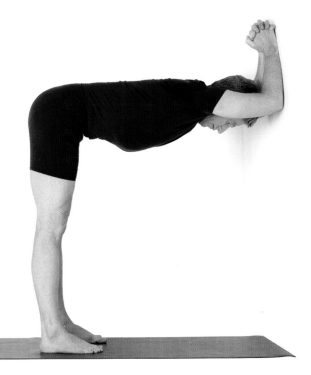

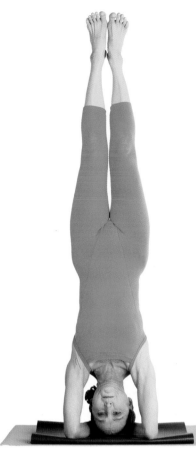

7.21
Salamba Sirsasana

SALAMBA SIRSASANA
HEADSTAND

PROPS
• set up as determined in Chapter 2

In this variation of Salamba Sirsasana (Figure 7.21), lift the bottom tips of your shoulder blades away from your elbows to avoid overarching your back.

Come into Salamba Sirsasana as described in Chapter 2. Make sure that your elbows are directly in line with your shoulder joints, so that your upper arms are parallel to each other. If your elbows are too far apart, your weight will fall onto your inner elbows. If your elbows are too close together, your weight will fall onto your outer elbows. When your elbows are properly aligned, the weight of your arms is evenly distributed between your inner and outer elbows.

In Salamba Sirsasana, let your rib cage rest back against your shoulder blades, and release the top edges of your shoulder blades away from your spine. Then lengthen from your outer armpits to your inner elbows. At the same time, lift the bottom tips of your shoulder blades away from your elbows to bring more weight onto your wrists.

Remain in Salamba Sirsasana for 3 to 5 minutes. Lift your inner triceps away from your inner elbows, and let them make contact with the bones of your upper arms. Where your inner triceps are firm against the bone, the muscle is strong; where your inner triceps drop away from the bone, the muscle is weak. Adjust your inner triceps so that they press evenly on your right and left arms. Then broaden your inner armpits, and lengthen your outer triceps down to your outer elbows.

To come out of the pose, lengthen your outer armpits and press your inner elbows into the floor as you lower your legs. Rest in Adho Mukha Virasana (Child's Pose, Figure 3.11b).

RELATED POSES. Pincha Mayurasana, Viparita Dandasana

SALAMBA SARVANGASANA
SHOULDERSTAND

PROPS
- set up as determined in Chapter 1

This variation of Salamba Sarvangasana (Figure 7.22) focuses on balancing your inner and outer triceps to bring your arms parallel with the sides of your rib cage.

Come into Salamba Sarvangasana as described in Chapter 1. If your elbows are not in firm contact with your blanket, place a folded mat under your elbows. If your weight falls onto your inner elbows and your arms slide away from your rib cage, use a strap above your elbows to keep your upper arms parallel. If your weight falls onto your outer elbows, your strap is too tight, and you may strain your neck. Adjust the strap so that your inner and outer elbows are in even contact with your blanket or support.

In Salamba Sarvangasana, relax your shoulders and widen your collarbones. Broaden your inner armpits and lengthen your outer triceps from your outer shoulders to your outer elbows. At the same time, lengthen from your outer armpits to your inner elbows, and lift your shoulder blades away from the floor.

Remain in Salamba Sarvangasana for 3 to 10 minutes. Lengthen your outer triceps toward your outer elbows, and lift your inner triceps away from the floor. As your inner triceps lift away from the floor, let your upper arm bones press down so that your weight rests on your bones and not on your muscles. Lift the bottom tips of your shoulder blades away from your elbows.

When you are ready to come out of the pose, release your inner groins and lower your legs into Halasana (Figure 3.17). Remain in Halasana for 1 to 3 minutes, adjusting your triceps and elbows as in Salamba Sarvangasana.

RELATED POSES. Halasana, Setu Bandhasana

7.22
Salamba Sarvangasana

PASCHIMOTTANASANA WITH HANDS ON BLOCKS
SITTING FORWARD BEND VARIATION

PROPS
- 1 nonskid mat
- 1 blanket or wedge
- 2 blocks

OPTIONAL PROP
- 1 chair

This variation of Paschimottanasana with Hands on Blocks (Figure 7.23) uses blocks under the hands to firm the elbows, open the shoulders, and lengthen the sides of the chest.

Place a folded blanket or wedge on your mat. Then sit at the edge of the blanket or wedge with your legs extended. Place two blocks by your outer feet. Lay the blocks flat if you are more flexible, or stand them on end if you are less flexible. (If you have tight hamstrings or problems with your lower back, use the seat of a chair, instead of blocks, to support your hands.) Extend your arms out to the sides with your palms facing up. With an inhalation, keep your elbows in line with the sides of your waist as you raise your arms overhead. With an exhalation, lift your kidneys away from your inner groins, and lengthen your torso over your thighs. Place your hands on the blocks with your arms extended.

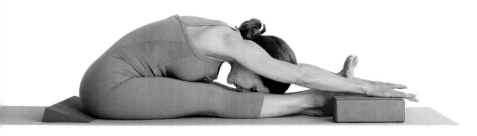

7.23
*Paschimottanasana
with Hands on Blocks*

In Paschimottanasana with Hands on Blocks, draw your inner groins away from your kidneys, and release your kidneys deeper into your body. Lengthen from your outer armpits to your inner elbows, and lift your inner elbows to firm your inner triceps. At the same time, stretch from your outer elbows to the mounds of your thumbs, and slide your hands forward on the blocks to lengthen the sides of your chest.

Remain in this position for 1 to 2 minutes. Broaden your inner armpits and lengthen your outer triceps as you bring your midsternum closer to your thighs. Keep your elbow joints firm, but release your shoulders and lengthen the sides of your chest.

To come out of the pose, keep your arms extended and slide your blocks back until your fingertips are in line with your knees and your torso is erect. Then place your hands by the sides of your hips, and return to an upright sitting position.

RELATED POSES. Janu Sirsasana, other sitting forward bends

Ujjayi Pranayama Sitting
Basic Yoga Breathing

Props
- 1 nonskid mat
- 1 blanket
- 1 wedge

Optional Props
- 1 or 2 blocks or blankets

This variation of Ujjayi Pranayama Sitting, with your hands resting on a wedge, demonstrates how the strength of your arms contributes to the fullness of your breath.

Rest in Savasana (Figure 3.22) for 2 to 3 minutes before you begin your breathing practice. Then sit on your mat at the edge of a folded blanket in your most comfortable sitting position: Padmasana with Hands on a Wedge (Lotus Pose Variation, Figure 7.24), Siddhasana (Perfect Pose, Figure 4.23), Sukhasana (Easy Pose, Figure 6.22), or Virasana (Hero Pose, Figure 5.24). If your knees are not in contact with the floor, use blocks or blankets to support them.

Lay a wedge across your feet or thighs with the thin edge pointing toward your pelvis. Align your elbows with the sides of your waist so that your upper arms are parallel with your back rib cage. Then place your hands on the wedge with your palms down. With an inhalation, firm your inner elbows and broaden your inner armpits as you lower your chin toward your sternal notch. With an exhalation, draw your eyes deeper into their sockets.

Begin with a deep, soft exhalation. With each inhalation, broaden your inner armpits, firm your inner elbows, and gently press your palms into the wedge. Allow

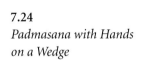

7.24

Padmasana with Hands on a Wedge

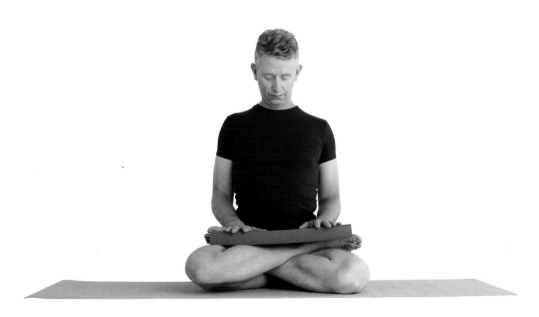

your breath to lift the front of your rib cage and uncoil your spine as if you were doing Urdhva Mukha Svanasana (Figure 7.17). With each exhalation, keep your inner elbows firm to stabilize your upper body and deepen your out breath.

Continue this cycle for 3 to 5 minutes. Then return to normal breathing, change the cross of your legs, and repeat this cycle for an equal length of time.

SAVASANA WITH ARMS SUPPORTED
RELAXATION POSE VARIATION

PROPS
- 1 nonskid mat
- 2 hand towels

OPTIONAL PROPS
- 1 to 3 blankets

7.25
Savasana with Arms Supported

In Savasana with Arms Supported (Figure 7.25), your forearms and elbows are supported by hand towels or folded blankets to help relax your shoulders.

Lie on your back on your nonskid mat with your arms and legs extended. (Place a folded blanket under your head and neck, if it feels more comfortable.) Then observe how your elbows and hands rest on the floor. If your arms are too close to your rib cage, your inner elbows and outer hands will press into the floor. If your arms are too far away from your rib cage, your outer elbows and inner hands will touch the floor.

Find the distance where you are balanced between your inner and outer elbows, and the back of your hands rest on the floor. Then take two hand towels, folding each of them first in half, and then in thirds. Place the folded towels under your forearms and elbows so that your elbows are raised from the floor. (If you need a higher lift, use folded blankets instead of hand towels.)

Remain in Savasana with Arms Supported for 5 to 10 minutes. With each inhalation, feel your shoulder blades widen. With each exhalation, relax the weight of your arms and shoulders. To come out of the pose, bend your knees and turn onto your side for a few breaths before pushing up with your hands.

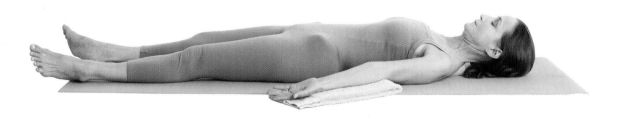

▶ PRACTICE SEQUENCE

TADASANA

URDHVA HASTASANA I

ARDHA UTTANASANA WITH HANDS ON THE WALL

ADHO MUKHA SVANASANA WITH HANDS ON BLOCKS

VIRABHADRASANA II

UTTANASANA WITH HANDS ON A BLOCK

UTTHITA PARSVAKONASANA WITH A BLOCK

PADANGUSTHASANA

VIRABHADRASANA I

ADHO MUKHA SVANASANA

VASISTHASANA

ADHO MUKHA VRKSASANA AT THE WALL

URDHVA MUKHA SVANASANA

URDHVA DHANURASANA WITH HANDS ON A WEDGE

BHARADVAJASANA II

ARDHA SIRSASANA WITH FOREARMS ON THE WALL

SALAMBA SIRSASANA

SALAMBA SARVANGASANA

HALASANA

PASCHIMOTTANASANA WITH HANDS ON BLOCKS

UJJAYI PRANAYAMA SITTING

SAVASANA WITH ARMS SUPPORTED

8 STRENGTHEN THE BASE OF YOUR NECK

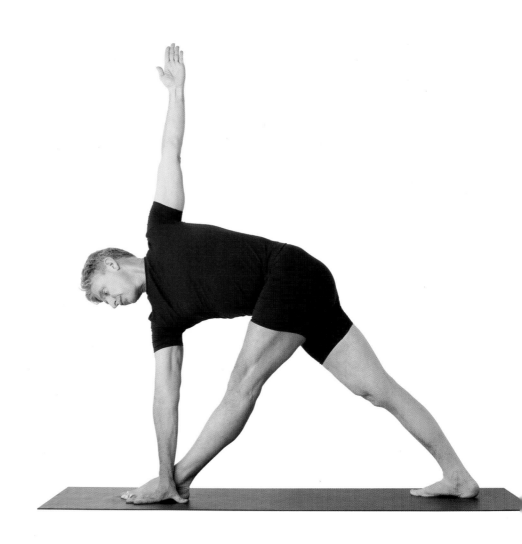

Long before babies begin to crawl, and even before they can roll from back to front, or from front to back, they must learn to lift their heads. Their heads are very large in proportion to the rest of their body, so this is an extraordinary achievement. In the photo of John Lyndon Griffin, my grandson, taken at the age of five months, you can see how his head is beautifully balanced and his shoulders completely relaxed. He holds his head erect from the core of his body (Figure 8.1).

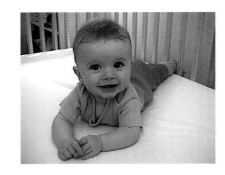

By the time you arrive at your first yoga class, you may have lost this instinctual alignment. Your head projects forward, your upper back rounds, and your shoulders hunch. You may feel stiffness and discomfort in the neck or be visited by periodic headaches. The muscles that form the ridge of your shoulders (the upper trapezius) sometimes ache with holding so much tension. You feel the weight of the world is on your shoulders, but you don't know how to let go.

The remedy this chapter offers is to strengthen the deeper muscles of the neck and upper thoracic (the splenius muscles), whose primary function is to extend the cervical spine and hold the head erect. The splenius muscles lie directly beneath the trapezius, and are composed of the splenius capitis and splenius cervicus. The splenius capitis originates from the nuchal ligament at the center of the neck and the spinous processes of C7–T3, and inserts at the base of the skull. The splenius cervicus runs from the spinous processes of T3–6 to the transverse processes of C1–3, and lies parallel to the splenius capitis (Figure 8.2).

8.1
John Lyndon Griffin

below:
8.2
The Splenius and Trapezius Muscles

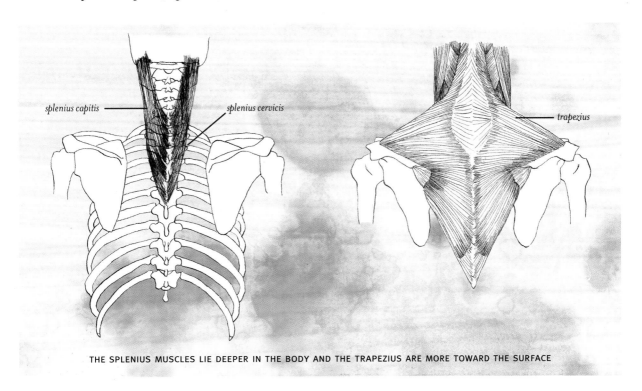

splenius capitis   *splenius cervicis*   *trapezius*

THE SPLENIUS MUSCLES LIE DEEPER IN THE BODY AND THE TRAPEZIUS ARE MORE TOWARD THE SURFACE

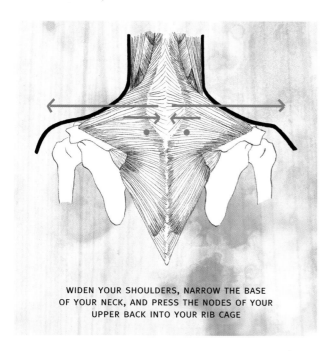

WIDEN YOUR SHOULDERS, NARROW THE BASE
OF YOUR NECK, AND PRESS THE NODES OF YOUR
UPPER BACK INTO YOUR RIB CAGE

above:
8.3
*The Nodes
of the Upper Back*

right:
8.4
*The Spines
of the Spine*

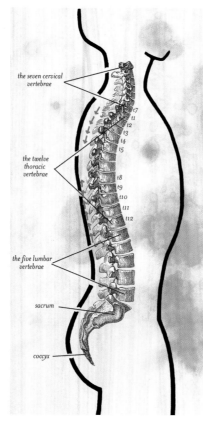

the seven cervical
vertebrae

c7
t1
t2
t3
t4
t5

the twelve
thoracic
vertebrae

t8
t9
t10
t11
t12

the five lumbar
vertebrae

sacrum

coccyx

In significant ways, the splenius muscles and the upper trapezius act as antagonists, that is, their actions counterbalance each other. Observe how the splenius muscles form an upright V, whereas the upper trapezius forms an inverted V. In other words, the fibers of the splenius muscles run in the opposite direction to the fibers of the upper trapezius. In practical terms, when the splenius muscles move in toward the spine, the upper trapezius releases away from the spine.

The instruction you will encounter later in this chapter, "Widen your shoulders, but narrow the muscles at the base of your neck," reflects this relationship. When you activate, or narrow, the splenius muscles at the base of your neck, you feel a spontaneous release, or widening, of the trapezius muscles that form the ridge of your shoulders. In this case, the strength of the deeper muscles of the body allows the surface muscles to relax (Figure 8.3).

To strengthen and protect the neck, the base of the neck is even more important than the neck itself. The neck is like the trunk of a tree and the base of the neck like its roots. The muscles at the base of your neck provide the foundation for the neck itself. For the trunk of your neck to lift upward, the muscles at the base of your neck must move down from the spine of C7 to the spine of T6.

Each vertebra of the spinal column is composed of a central body, a transverse process on either side, and a spinous process projecting directly back. For the sake of convenience, I refer to the spinous processes as "the spines of the spine." If you look at a drawing of the spinal column in profile, you will notice that the spines project at different angles. The spines of the lower thoracic point more downward, while the spines of the upper thoracic point more outward (Figure 8.4).

If you pull your lower thoracic spines down even farther, you will eventually overarch your back by gripping and tightening that portion of your spine. In Tadasana (Figure 8.6), Adho Mukha Svanasana (Figure 8.14), and especially in backbends, let your lower thoracic spines move away from one another—that is, up toward your head—to create space between your lower thoracic vertebrae.

If your upper back is rounded and your upper thoracic spines protrude, your splenius muscles are not providing adequate support. To strengthen the base of your neck, start with your C7, where the spine is most prominent. Standing in Tadasana, lift the body of C7 up toward your head, and turn the spine of C7 down toward the spine of T1. As you draw the spine of C7 down, lift up from the base of your skull to lengthen the back of your neck. Then, sequentially, turn the spine of T1 down toward the spine of T2, and the spine of T2 down toward the spine of T3.

To stabilize your upper back as you make these adjustments, press the nodes of your upper back into your body. The nodes of your upper back are two pressure points located just inside the inner corners of your shoulder blades, in line with the sides of your neck. Keep the nodes of your upper back in firm contact with your back rib cage to prevent squeezing your shoulder blades together too much or pulling them too far apart.

If your upper back is flat or concave, you may be gripping and squeezing your upper thoracic spine. In this case, press the nodes of your upper back into your body, but keep your upper thoracic vertebrae wide as you draw the spine of C7 gently down. You want to strengthen the muscles at the base of the neck and make them more resilient, not tighten them.

Remember that the shape of your cervical spine (C1–C7) is a mirror image of your upper thoracic spine (T1–T6). If your upper thoracic spine is flat, the curve of your cervical spine will be flat or even reversed. If your upper thoracic curve is overly rounded, your cervical curve will be overly arched. When your upper thoracic vertebrae are properly aligned, your neck will maintain its natural, healthy curve (Figure 8.5).

8.5
Adjusting Your Cervical Curve

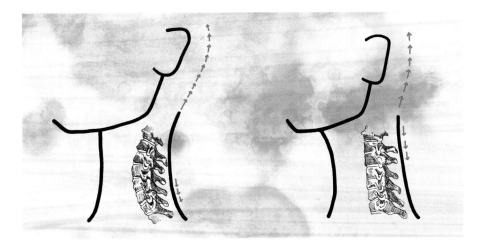

TADASANA
MOUNTAIN POSE

PROP
• 1 nonskid mat

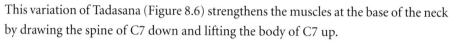

This variation of Tadasana (Figure 8.6) strengthens the muscles at the base of the neck by drawing the spine of C7 down and lifting the body of C7 up.

Stand on your mat in Tadasana with your feet together and your arms extended by your sides. Adjust your pelvis so that your inner groins are in line with your kidneys, and lift your kidneys away from your inner groins. Relax your collarbones and widen your shoulders, but narrow the muscles at the base of your neck.

In Tadasana, adjust your head and neck so that your inner ears are directly in line with the center of your shoulder joints. Then lift the base of your skull, and draw the spine of C7 toward the spine of T1. Press the nodes of your upper back into your rib cage, and draw the spine of T1 toward the spine of T2. Finally, lift the spines of your lower thoracic toward your midthoracic as you draw the spine of T2 toward the spine of T3. Keep your midsternum wide.

8.6
Tadasana

Maintain this position for several breaths. Lift up from the base of your skull and draw the spine of C7 down to lengthen the back of your neck. Return to Tadasana between each of the standing poses to adjust your head and neck.

Practice Notes. If you have a flat or reversed cervical curve, draw the spines of your *upper* cervical vertebrae (C1–3) toward the middle of your neck to restore a natural curve. If your neck is overarched and needs to be lengthened, draw the spines of your *lower* cervical vertebrae (C4–6) toward C7. If your sixth cervical vertebra is deeply set into your body, focus on turning the spine of C6 toward the spine of C7 (Figure 8.5).

VIRABHADRASANA II
WARRIOR POSE II

PROP
- 1 nonskid mat

This variation of Virabhadrasana II (Figure 8.7) strengthens the muscles at the base of your neck by aligning the cervical and thoracic spines.

Stand on your mat in Tadasana (Figure 8.6), and separate your legs approximately 4½ feet apart. Turn your left foot in 30 degrees and your right foot out 90 degrees. Bring your inner groins in line with your kidneys and lengthen your spine. With an inhalation, press the nodes of your upper back into your rib cage as you raise your arms out to the sides to shoulder level. With an exhalation, turn your head to look over your right hand as you bend your right knee to form a square.

In Virabhadrasana II, lift your kidneys away from your inner groins. Widen your midsternum and lengthen from your outer armpits to your inner elbows. As you turn your head to the right, let your chin drop toward your right collarbone, and lift the base of your skull toward the crown of your head. At the same time, turn the body of your C7 toward the left, so that your rib cage faces directly forward. Then relax your collarbones, widen your sternal notch, and let the nodes of your upper back move deeper into your body to stabilize your head and neck.

8.7
Virabhadrasana II

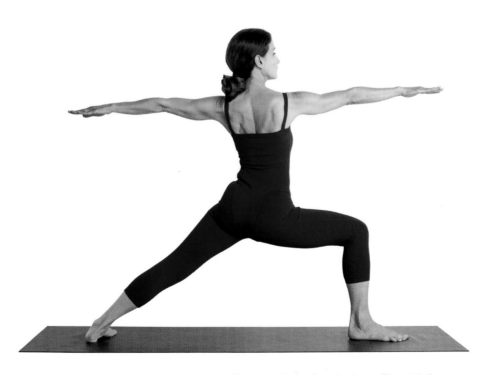

Maintain this position for 30 seconds. Widen your shoulders, but narrow the base of your neck. Draw the spine of C7 toward the spine of T1, the spine of T1 toward the spine of T2, and the spine of T2 toward the spine of T3. At the same time, lift the spines of your lower thoracic toward your midthoracic, and keep your midsternum broad.

To come out of the pose, lift up from your C7 as you straighten your bent leg with an inhalation and lower your arms with an exhalation. Then repeat to the other side.

RELATED POSE. Ardha Chandrasana

ARDHA CHANDRASANA
HALF-MOON POSE

8.8
Ardha Chandrasana

PROP
• 1 nonskid mat

OPTIONAL PROP
• 1 block

This variation of Ardha Chandrasana (Figure 8.8), with your head looking down at the floor, strengthens the muscles at the base of your neck and improves your balance.

Stand on your mat in Tadasana (Figure 8.6), and separate your legs approximately 4 feet apart. Turn your left foot in 30 degrees and your right foot out 90 degrees. With an inhalation, press the nodes of your upper back into your body as you raise your arms out to the side to shoulder level. With an exhalation, bend your right knee over

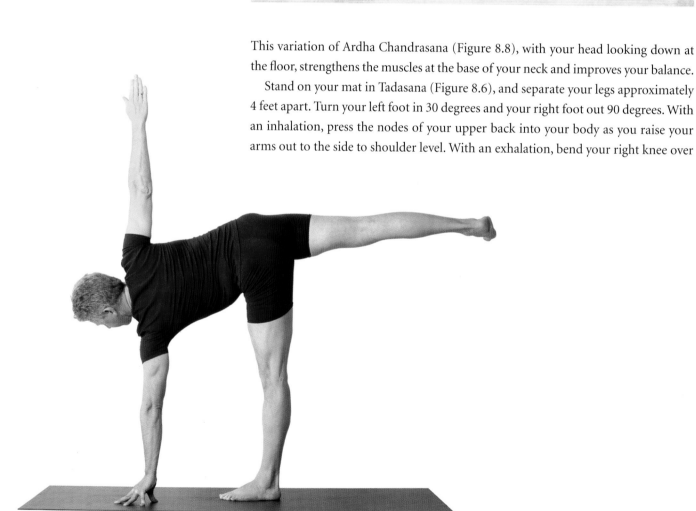

your right foot, come up onto the toes of your left foot, and place the fingertips of your right hand on the floor directly under your right shoulder. (If you cannot reach the floor easily, use a block under your right hand.) With another inhalation, turn your head and neck to look directly at the floor. With an exhalation, lift your right thighbone to straighten your right leg.

In Ardha Chandrasana, bring your inner groins in line with your kidneys, and lengthen your kidneys away from your inner groins. Turn your head to look down at the floor, and, at the same time, turn the body of your C7 toward the ceiling. Then lengthen from your outer armpits to your inner elbows, press the nodes of your upper back deeper into your body, and turn the spine of C7 toward the spine of T1.

Maintain this position for 30 seconds. Widen your shoulders, turn your head toward the floor, and narrow the muscles at the base of your neck. If you tend to arch your back, let your lower thoracic spines move toward your midthoracic vertebrae, but continue to draw the spine of C7 toward the spine of T1.

To come out of the pose, lengthen your right arm with an inhalation to stabilize your upper body, and, with an exhalation, bend your right knee and lower your left leg to the floor. Repeat to the other side.

RELATED POSES. Utthita Trikonasana, Parivrtta Trikonasana, Parivrtta Ardha Chandrasana, Utthita Parsvakonasana

8.9
Uttanasana

UTTANASANA
STANDING FORWARD BEND

PROP
• 1 nonskid mat

OPTIONAL PROP
• 1 block

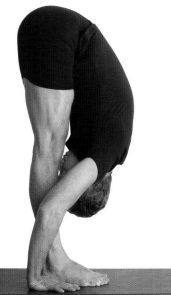

This variation of Uttanasana (Figure 8.9) relaxes the muscles at the base of the neck and releases the cervical spine.

Stand on your mat in Tadasana (Figure 8.6) with your feet a few inches apart, and place your hands on your hips with your thumbs pressing down on the top edge of your sacrum. With an inhalation, lift your kidneys away from your inner groins. With an exhalation, draw your groins into your body as you lengthen your torso forward. Then place your hands on the floor by the sides of your feet, relax your shoulders, and let your head hang freely. (If your hands don't reach the floor easily, use a block to support them.)

In Uttanasana, lift your groins away from your kidneys, and release your kidneys away from your groins to lengthen your abdomen. Create space between your lower thoracic spines by moving them toward your midthoracic vertebrae. Widen your midsternum and create space between your midthoracic vertebrae. Firm your inner elbows, press the nodes of your upper back into your body, and widen the muscles at the base of your neck.

Now work, vertebra by vertebra, to release your upper thoracic spine and lengthen your neck. Move the spine of T3 toward the spine of T2, the spine of T2 toward the spine of T1, and the spine of T1 toward the spine of C7. Then move the spine of C7 toward the spine of C6, and the spine of C6 toward the spine of C5. Move the hollows at the base of your skull toward the crown of your head and deepen your sternal notch.

Maintain this position for 1 minute. Firm your inner elbows, press the nodes of your upper back into your body, and widen the base of your neck. Let your eyes rest deep in their sockets.

To come out of the pose, lift your head, turn the spine of C7 toward the spine of T1, and place your hands on your hips. With an inhalation, lift your torso from the strength of your upper thoracic spine. With an exhalation, return to Tadasana.

RELATED POSE. Prasarita Padottanasana (Phase 2)

8.10
Utthita Trikonasana

UTTHITA TRIKONASANA
EXTENDED TRIANGLE POSE

PROP
• 1 nonskid mat

OPTIONAL PROP
• 1 block

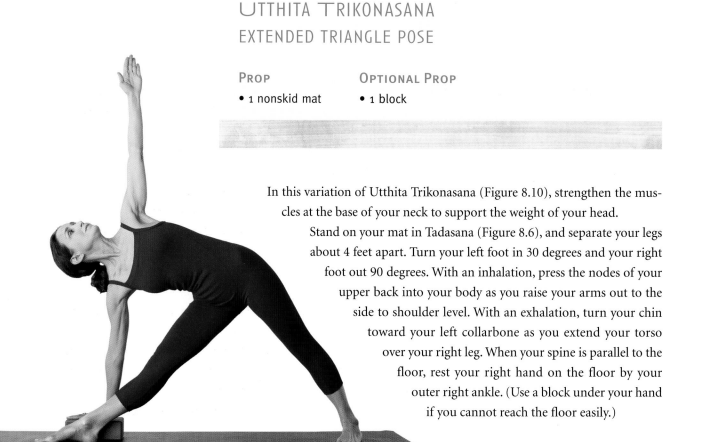

In this variation of Utthita Trikonasana (Figure 8.10), strengthen the muscles at the base of your neck to support the weight of your head.

Stand on your mat in Tadasana (Figure 8.6), and separate your legs about 4 feet apart. Turn your left foot in 30 degrees and your right foot out 90 degrees. With an inhalation, press the nodes of your upper back into your body as you raise your arms out to the side to shoulder level. With an exhalation, turn your chin toward your left collarbone as you extend your torso over your right leg. When your spine is parallel to the floor, rest your right hand on the floor by your outer right ankle. (Use a block under your hand if you cannot reach the floor easily.)

In Utthita Trikonasana, check that your inner groins are in line with your kidneys, and lift your kidneys away from your inner groins. Firm your inner elbows, press the nodes of your upper back into your body, and turn the spine of T1 toward the spine of T2. Then widen your collarbones, turn the spine of C7 toward the spine of T1, and let your head drop back. Keep your eyes soft and your spine long.

Maintain this position for 1 minute. Widen your shoulders and relax the sides of your neck, but narrow the muscles at the base of your neck. Let your head hang freely.

To come out of the pose, first lower your chin toward your left collarbone so that your neck is in a neutral position. Then, with an inhalation, lift your torso to a vertical position, and, with an exhalation, lower your arms. Repeat to the other side.

Practice Notes. If you have a weak or injured neck, turn your head to face the floor as in the preceding variation of Ardha Chandrasana (Figure 8.8).

8.11
Parivrtta Trikonasana

RELATED POSE. Utthita Parsvakonasana

PARIVRTTA TRIKONASANA
REVOLVED TRIANGLE POSE

PROP
• 1 nonskid mat

OPTIONAL PROP
• 1 block

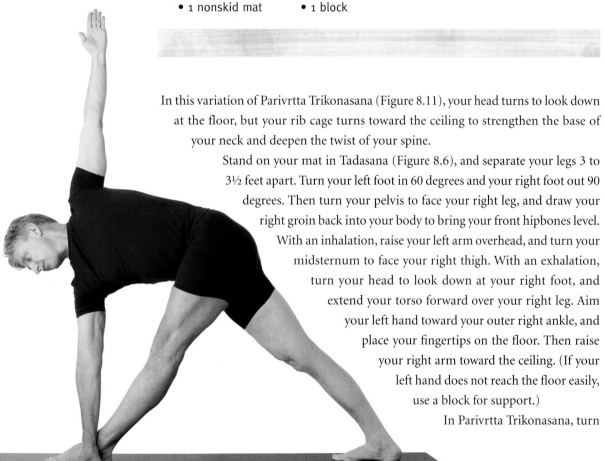

In this variation of Parivrtta Trikonasana (Figure 8.11), your head turns to look down at the floor, but your rib cage turns toward the ceiling to strengthen the base of your neck and deepen the twist of your spine.

Stand on your mat in Tadasana (Figure 8.6), and separate your legs 3 to 3½ feet apart. Turn your left foot in 60 degrees and your right foot out 90 degrees. Then turn your pelvis to face your right leg, and draw your right groin back into your body to bring your front hipbones level. With an inhalation, raise your left arm overhead, and turn your midsternum to face your right thigh. With an exhalation, turn your head to look down at your right foot, and extend your torso forward over your right leg. Aim your left hand toward your outer right ankle, and place your fingertips on the floor. Then raise your right arm toward the ceiling. (If your left hand does not reach the floor easily, use a block for support.)

In Parivrtta Trikonasana, turn

your head and neck to look down at the floor, and, simultaneously, turn your rib cage and the body of your C7 toward the ceiling. (This action will deepen your twist and improve your balance.) Then widen your shoulders, narrow the base of your neck, and draw the spine of C7 toward the spine of T1.

Maintain this position for about 1 minute. If you are a beginner or if you have problems with your neck, continue to look down at the floor. If you are more experienced and your neck is strong, turn your chin from your left collarbone toward your right collarbone, and then let your head drop back, supported by the muscles at the base of your neck.

To come out of the pose, first, lift your chin toward your right collarbone; then turn it toward your left collarbone, so that your head once again faces the floor. With an inhalation, lift your torso from the strength of your upper thoracic spine. With an exhalation, return to Tadasana. Repeat to the other side.

RELATED POSE. Parivrtta Ardha Chandrasana

8.12
Padangusthasana

PADANGUSTHASANA
TOE-HOLDING POSE

PROP
• 1 nonskid mat

OPTIONAL PROP
• 1 block

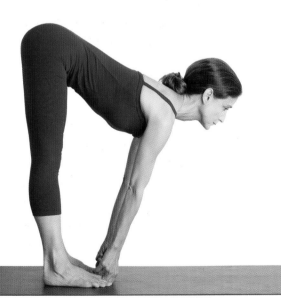

This variation of Padangusthasana (Figure 8.12) strengthens the muscles at the base of the neck and lengthens the spine.

Stand on your mat in Tadasana (Figure 8.6) with your feet a few inches apart. Place your hands on your hips with your thumbs pressing down on the top edge of your sacrum. Widen your collarbones, firm your inner elbows, and press the nodes of your upper back into your body. With an inhalation, lift your kidneys away from your inner groins. Turn the spine of C7 toward the spine of T1, and let your head drop back. With an exhalation, release your groins and lengthen your torso forward. Keep your head lifted and your eyes soft. When your spine is parallel to the floor, extend your arms and wrap your second and third fingers around your big toes. (If you are unable to reach your feet without rounding your back, place a block on end in front of your feet, and rest your hands on the block.)

In Padangusthasana, lengthen your kidneys away from your inner groins, and move your inner groins away from your kidneys. Firm your inner elbows, press the nodes of your upper back into your body, and lift your head from the base of your skull. At the same time, relax the sides of your neck, and turn the spine of C7 toward the spine of T1. Then lift your lower thoracic spines toward your midthoracic vertebrae, but turn the spine of T1 toward the spine of T2, and the spine of T2 toward the spine of T3. Relax the sides of your respiratory diaphragm.

Maintain this position for 30 seconds. With an inhalation, widen your shoulders but narrow the base of your neck. With an exhalation, draw the spine of C7 toward the spine of T1 as you lengthen your spinal column.

To come out of the pose, place your hands on your hips, and lift your torso from the strength of your upper thoracic spine. Then straighten your arms and return to Tadasana.

8.13

Virabhadrasana I

RELATED POSE. Prasarita Padottanasana (Phase 1)

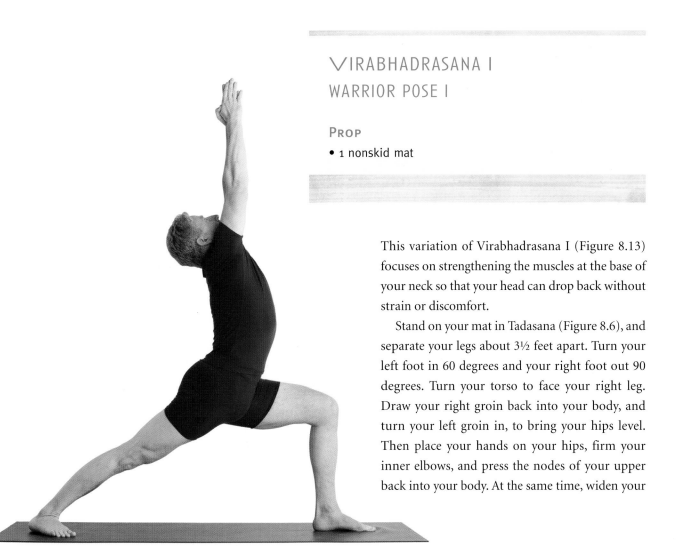

VIRABHADRASANA I
WARRIOR POSE I

PROP
• 1 nonskid mat

This variation of Virabhadrasana I (Figure 8.13) focuses on strengthening the muscles at the base of your neck so that your head can drop back without strain or discomfort.

Stand on your mat in Tadasana (Figure 8.6), and separate your legs about 3½ feet apart. Turn your left foot in 60 degrees and your right foot out 90 degrees. Turn your torso to face your right leg. Draw your right groin back into your body, and turn your left groin in, to bring your hips level. Then place your hands on your hips, firm your inner elbows, and press the nodes of your upper back into your body. At the same time, widen your collarbones and let your head drop back. (If your neck is vulnerable to injury, keep your head erect or practice with a partner supporting the base of your skull.) With an inhalation, lift your kidneys away from your inner groins as you raise your arms overhead. With an exhalation, bend your right knee to form a square.

In Virabhadrasana I, lift your kidneys away from your inner groins, and lengthen from your outer armpits to your inner elbows. Widen your midsternum, relax the sides of your neck, and lift your C7 deeper into your body. If the spine of C7 moves to the right or the left of your spinal column, draw it gently toward the median line of your body. Then draw the spine of C7 toward the spine of T1, and press the nodes of your upper back into your body.

Maintain this position for 30 seconds. Lift your arms from the strength of your inner elbows, widen your shoulders, and narrow the base of your neck. Gently turn the spine of C7 toward the spine of T1, and let your eyes rest deep in their sockets.

To come out of the pose, straighten your bent leg with an inhalation, and lower your arms with an exhalation. Repeat to the other side.

ADHO MUKHA SVANASANA
DOWNWARD-FACING DOG POSE

PROP
• 1 nonskid mat

8.14
Adho Mukha Svanasana

In this variation of Adho Mukha Svanasana (Figure 8.14), come into the pose with your head lifted to strengthen the muscles at the base of your neck; then let your head drop down to relax your neck completely.

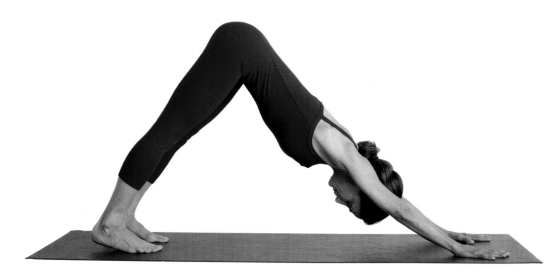

Start on your hands and knees on your mat, with the mounds of your thumbs in line with the center of your shoulder joints and your pelvis over your knees. Turn your elbow creases to face your thumbs, lift your rib cage away from your inner elbows, and curl your toes under. With an inhalation, lift your head from the base of your skull, and turn the spine of C7 toward the spine of T1. With an exhalation, lift your pelvis, straighten your legs, and lengthen the sides of your chest. Keep your head lifted until your ears are in line with your upper arms; then let your head drop down, and relax the sides of your neck.

In Adho Mukha Svanasana, move your groins away from your kidneys and lengthen your kidneys. At the same time, lift your lower thoracic spines toward your midthoracic vertebrae to lengthen your spinal column. Widen your midsternum and create space between your midthoracic vertebrae. Then firm your inner elbows, press the nodes of your upper back into your rib cage, and widen the muscles at the base of your neck. Turn the spine of T2 toward the spine of T1, and the spine of T1 toward the spine of C7. Then turn the spine of C7 toward the spine of C6 and deepen your sternal notch. Relax the hollows at the base of your skull.

Maintain this position for 1 to 2 minutes. Firm your inner elbows and lengthen the sides of your chest, but let your head hang freely from the muscles at the base of your neck. Bring the roof of your mouth parallel to the floor.

To come out of the pose, bend your knees, sit back on your heels, and rest for a few breaths in Adho Mukha Virasana (Child's Pose, Figure 3.11b).

8.15
*Pincha Mayurasana
at the Wall*

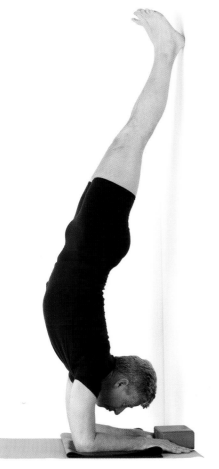

PINCHA MAYURASANA AT THE WALL
ELBOW BALANCE VARIATION

PROPS
- 1 nonskid mat
- 1 wall
- 1 block

OPTIONAL PROP
- 1 strap

In this variation of Pincha Mayurasana at the Wall (Figure 8.15), the head is lifted to strengthen the muscles at the base of the neck and activate the upper thoracic spine.

Place a nonskid mat folded in half or in quarters at the base of a wall. Put a block on the mat against the wall to separate and stabilize your hands. Then kneel in front of the mat, and position your hands so that your index fingers touch the sides of the block, your thumbs press the front edge of the block, and your palms lie flat. Place your elbows directly under the center of your shoulder joints, so that your forearms are parallel. (If your elbows slide away from each other, use a strap around your upper arms to hold them in place.)

Lift the sides of your rib cage away from your inner elbows, turn your toes under, and lift your pelvis to straighten your legs. With an inhalation, bend one leg and step the foot a few inches closer to the wall. With an exhalation, keep your other leg perfectly straight as you swing it in a wide arc toward the wall. Let the momentum of your straight leg draw your bent leg away from the floor. Then rest your heels on the wall with your legs extended, and lift your inner groins away from your kidneys.

In Pincha Mayurasana at the Wall, press the tips of your elbows into the floor and lengthen the sides of your rib cage, to open your shoulders. At the same time, press the nodes of your upper back into your body, and draw the spine of T2 toward the spine of T3, and the spine of T1 toward the spine of T2. Then widen your collarbones, turn your sternal notch toward the base of your throat, and draw the spine of C7 toward the spine of T1. To raise your head, turn the spine of C6 toward the spine of C7, and lift up from the hollows at the base of your skull.

Maintain this position for 30 seconds. Lift the sides of your rib cage away from your inner elbows. Broaden your sternal notch and turn the spine of C7 toward the spine of T1. If you have a shoulder imbalance, check that your cervical and upper thoracic spines are all aligned with the median line of your body.

To come out of the pose, press the nodes of your upper back into your rib cage, release your inner groins, and slowly lower your legs. Rest for several breaths in Adho Mukha Virasana (Child's Pose, Figure 3.11b).

Practice Notes. If you have tight shoulders or discomfort in your neck, do not raise your head, but let it hang between your upper arms, and focus on lengthening the sides of your rib cage.

RELATED POSE. Adho Mukha Vrksasana

8.16
Ustrasana

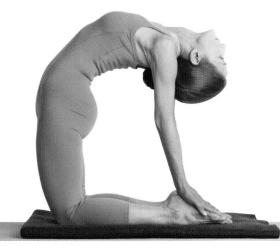

USTRASANA
CAMEL POSE

PROPS
- 1 nonskid mat
- 1 blanket

OPTIONAL PROPS
- 1 to 3 blocks
- 1 bolster

In this variation of Ustrasana (Figure 8.16), the upper thoracic spines draw down to strengthen the muscles at the base of the neck and allow the head to hang freely.

Place a folded blanket on top of your nonskid mat to protect your knees and shins. Then kneel on your blanket with your knees and

CAUTION

If you experience pain
or discomfort in your
neck in Ustrasana, do not
let your head drop back.
Either keep you head
lifted and your chin
tucked in to your chest
or work with a partner
supporting the base of
your skull.

feet in line with your hip joints. (You can use a block between your feet if they tend to slide together.) Place your hands on your hips with your thumbs pressing down on the top edge of your sacrum. With an inhalation, firm your inner elbows, press the nodes of your upper back into your body, and let your head drop back, but only if it feels comfortable on your neck. With an exhalation, lift your kidneys away from your inner groins, widen your midsternum, and extend your arms to take hold of your feet. (If you cannot reach your feet easily, use blocks to support your hands or place a bolster crosswise over your ankles.)

In Ustrasana, lengthen your inner groins away from your kidneys, and lift your kidneys away from your inner groins to lengthen your lumbar spine. Turn your elbow creases to face the mounds of your thumbs, firm your inner elbows, and press the nodes of your upper back into your body. At the same time, draw the spine of T2 toward the spine of T3, and the spine of T1 toward the spine of T2. Then widen your collarbones, deepen your sternal notch, and turn the spine of C7 toward the spine of T1.

Maintain this position for 30 seconds. To lengthen the curve of your neck, draw the spine of C6 toward the spine of C7, and the spine of C5 toward the spine of C6. At the same time, press the base of your skull away from the back of your neck. Check that your cervical and upper thoracic spines are aligned with the median line of your body.

To come out of Ustrasana, bend your elbows and place your hands on your hips. With an inhalation, press your knees into the floor, draw your inner groins back into your body, and lift your torso from the strength of your upper thoracic spine. With an exhalation, sit back on your heels. Repeat this pose two or three times.

RELATED POSES. Urdhva Mukha Svanasana, Salabhasana, Urdhva Dhanurasana, other backbends

CAUTION

If you have problems
with your neck, practice
Urdhva Dhanurasana
Figure 3.13) instead
of Viparita Dandasana
with Feet on a Chair.

VIPARITA DANDASANA WITH FEET ON A CHAIR
INVERTED STAFF POSE VARIATION

PROPS
- 1 nonskid mat
- 1 chair

- 1 wall

OPTIONAL PROPS
- 2 folded mats or blankets

This variation of Viparita Dandasana with Feet on a Chair (Figure 8.17), with the head lifted, strengthens the muscles at the base of the neck and mobilizes the upper thoracic spine.

Place the back legs of your chair against a wall. Lay a nonskid mat lengthwise in front of the chair to provide a cushion for your head and forearms. Then lie on your back with your buttocks under the seat of the chair and your lower legs resting on the chair. Raise your arms overhead and place your hands on the floor by your outer shoulders with your palms flat. With an inhalation, place the soles of your feet on the seat of the chair and lift your pelvis. With an exhalation, press down with your hands and lift onto the crown on your head. Place one forearm at a time on your mat, and interlock your hands behind your head as for Salamba Sirsasana (Figure 8.19). Then press your forearms into the mat, and lift your head away from the floor. (If you cannot lift your head because your arms are short or your shoulders are tight, use folded mats or blankets under your forearms to give yourself an extra lift.)

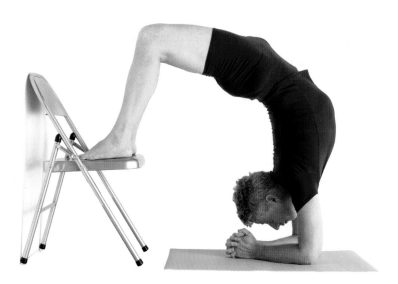

8.17
*Viparita Dandasana
with Feet on a Chair*

In Viparita Dandasana with Feet on a Chair, lengthen your inner groins away from your kidneys, and lift your kidneys away from your inner groins. Turn your sternal notch toward the base of your throat, and lift your head from the base of your skull so that you are facing the floor. Lift the sides of your rib cage away from your inner elbows, and press the nodes of your upper back into your body. Draw the spine of C7 toward the spine of T1.

Maintain this position for 1 minute. Widen your shoulders, but narrow the base of your neck. Check that your cervical and upper thoracic spines are aligned with the median line of your body. Draw the spine of C6 toward the spine of C7 to lift your head higher and lengthen your cervical spine.

To come out of the pose, first, place the crown of your head on the floor. Then release the clasp of your hands, place your palms flat on the floor, and lower your torso. Rest with your feet on the chair and your knees out to the side until your breathing returns to normal. Repeat two or three times.

RELATED POSE. Urdhva Dhanurasana

BHARADVAJASANA II
SIMPLE SEATED TWIST II

PROPS
- 1 nonskid mat
- 1 blanket

OPTIONAL PROPS
- 1 block or blanket
- 1 strap

This variation of Bharadvajasana II has an active phase and a restful phase. In the active phase (Figure 8.18a), your head turns in the opposite direction from your rib cage to lengthen the sides of your neck and release your cervical spine. In the restful phase (Figure 8.18b), the head and rib cage turn in the same direction, and the spinal column is more relaxed.

Place a folded blanket on your mat, and sit on the blanket with your legs extended. Bend your right leg into Virasana (Hero Pose, Figure 5.24), with the top of your right foot on the floor beside your outer right hip. Bring your left leg into Padmasana (Lotus Pose, Figure 3.21), with your left foot resting on your right thigh. (If you have knee problems or tight hip joints, place your left foot on the floor near your inner right thigh. Use a block or blanket to support your left knee, if your knee does not touch the floor.)

Place your fingertips on the floor beside your pelvis. With an inhalation, firm your inner elbows, widen your midsternum, and press the nodes of your upper back into your body. At the same time, turn your chin toward your right collarbone, and look

below left:
8.18a
Bharadvajasana II, Phase 1

below right:
8.18b
Bharadvajasana II, Phase 2

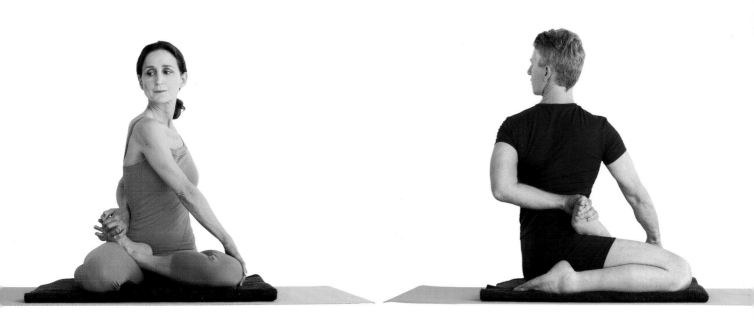

over your right shoulder. With an exhalation, bring your left forearm behind your back, and take hold of your left foot with your left hand. (Use a strap around your left ankle if you cannot reach your foot.) Then place the palm of your right hand on your outer left thigh.

Phase 1. In Bharadvajasana II, turn the body of your C7 toward the left, but turn your head and neck toward the right. Feel the stretch of the trapezius muscle along the left side of your neck and the ridge of your left shoulder. Then widen your collarbones away from your sternal notch, and draw the spine of C7 toward the spine of T1. Press the nodes of your upper back against your rib cage, and draw the spine of T1 toward the spine of T2. At the same time, lift from the base of your skull toward the crown of your head to lengthen the back of your neck. Maintain this position for two or three breaths.

Phase 2. With an exhalation, turn your head to look over your left shoulder, and drop your chin toward your left collarbone. Let your spinal column relax. Now broaden your midsternum and, without gripping, turn from your midthoracic vertebrae. Lift the spines of your lower thoracic vertebrae up toward your midthoracic; at the same time, draw the spines of C7, T1, and T2 gently down. Relax your shoulders and lift from the base of your skull. Find the quiet center of the pose. Then release your hold on your left foot, and repeat to the other side.

Practice Notes. To relieve a stiff neck, practice Bharadvajasana II and other sitting twists with your head turned in the opposite direction from your rib cage (Phase 1).

RELATED POSES. Other sitting twists

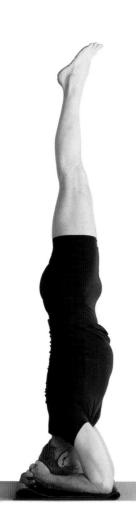

8.19
Salamba Sirsasana

SALAMBA SIRSASANA
HEADSTAND

PROPS
• set up as determined in Chapter 2

This variation of Salamba Sirsasana (Figure 8.19) focuses on maintaining a natural cervical curve by strengthening the muscles at the base of the neck.

Come into Salamba Sirsasana as described in Chapter 2. As you walk your feet in toward your blanket, turn your lower thoracic spines toward your midthoracic vertebrae to protect your neck and release your lower back. Then either bend your knees into your chest or come into the pose with your legs straight, depending on your strength and flexibility.

In Salamba Sirsasana, lift the sides of your rib cage away from your inner elbows and widen your collarbones. Release your shoulder blades away from your spine, but press the nodes of your upper back into your body to stabilize the base of your neck. Then turn the base of your skull away from the back of your neck, and press the crown of your head gently into your blanket. If you have a flat or reversed cervical curve, draw the spines of your *upper* cervical vertebrae (C1–3) toward the middle of your neck to restore a natural curve (Figure 8.5). If your neck is overarched and needs to be lengthened, draw the spines of your *lower* cervical vertebrae (C4–6) toward C7. If your sixth cervical vertebra is deeply set into your body, focus on turning the spine of C6 toward the spine of C7.

Maintain this position for 3 to 5 minutes. Move the base of your skull away from the back of your neck, and turn the spine of C7 toward the spine of T1. Then press the nodes of your upper back into your rib cage and firm your inner elbows. Turn the spine of T1 toward the spine of T2, and the spine of T2 toward the spine of T3. If your lower rib cage protrudes, turn the spines of your lower thoracic toward your midthoracic. Balance your spines to balance your body.

To come out of the pose, turn your lower thoracic spines toward your midthoracic vertebrae to release your lower back, and either bend your knees into your chest or come down with straight legs. Rest in Adho Mukha Virasana (Child's Pose, Figure 3.11b) until your breathing returns to normal.

8.20
Setu Bandhasana with Blocks under the Sacrum

SETU BANDHASANA WITH BLOCKS UNDER THE SACRUM
BRIDGE POSE VARIATION

PROPS
- 1 nonskid mat
- 1 blanket
- 2 blocks

OPTIONAL PROP
- 1 strap

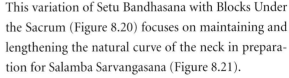

This variation of Setu Bandhasana with Blocks Under the Sacrum (Figure 8.20) focuses on maintaining and lengthening the natural curve of the neck in preparation for Salamba Sarvangasana (Figure 8.21).

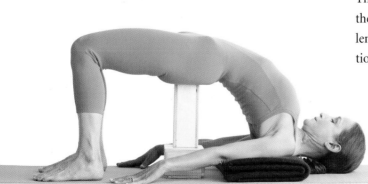

Take a standard folded blanket, and fold it in half again lengthwise. Put the blanket on a nonskid mat, and lie on your back with your shoulders at the folded edge of the blanket. Bend your knees, place the soles of your feet on the floor with your heels close to your sitting bones, and lift your pelvis. Set the first block flat on the floor beneath your pelvis, and the second block vertically on top of the first to support your lower sacrum and tailbone. (If you find if helpful, loop a strap around your wrists, extend your arms on the floor, and press out against the strap.)

In Setu Bandhasana with Blocks Under the Sacrum, widen your shoulders and lengthen from your outer armpits to your inner elbows. At the same time, press the nodes of your upper back into your body, and lift the sides of your rib cage. Then release your collarbones away from your sternal notch, and turn the spine of C7 toward the spine of T1. When you make this adjustment, feel how your C7 lifts away from the blanket, taking weight off your neck.

Remain in this position for 2 to 3 minutes. To lengthen your neck and bring your chin closer to your upper sternum, gently turn the base of your skull toward the crown of your head; simultaneously, draw the spines of your *lower* cervical vertebrae toward the base of your neck. (If you have a flat or reversed cervical curve, draw the spines of your *upper* cervical vertebrae toward the middle of your neck to restore a natural curve.) Soften your gaze and draw your eyes deeper into their sockets.

To come out of the pose, release your arms from the strap, lift your pelvis, take away the blocks, and rest your pelvis on the floor.

8.21
Salamba Sarvangasana

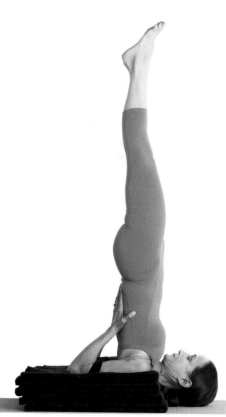

SALAMBA SARVANGASANA
SHOULDERSTAND

PROPS
- set up as determined in Chapter 1

This variation of Salamba Sarvangasana (Figure 8.21) strengthens the muscles at the base of the neck and takes weight off C7.

Come into Salamba Sarvangasana as described in Chapter 1. Place your hands on your back with your palms flat and your fingers pointing toward your waist.

In Salamba Sarvangasana, widen your shoulders and lengthen from your outer armpits to your inner elbows. At the same time, press the nodes of your upper back into your body, and lift the sides of your rib cage. Then release your collarbones away from your sternal notch, and turn the spine of C7 toward the spine of T1 and the spine of T1 toward the spine of T2. To lengthen your neck, turn from the base of your skull toward the crown of your head; simultaneously, draw the spines of your *lower* cervical vertebrae (C4–C6) toward the base of your neck (Figure 8.5). If you have a flat or reversed cervical curve, draw the spines of your *upper* cervical vertebrae (C1–C3) toward the middle of your neck to restore a natural curve.

Remain in this position for 3 to 10 minutes. If you have a shoulder imbalance, check that your cervical and upper thoracic spines are all aligned with the median line of your body, especially the spine of C7. Release the base of your skull away from the back of your neck, so that your inner ears feel open and round. Soften your gaze.

To come out of the pose, release your inner groins and lower your legs into Halasana (Figure 3.17). In Halasana, follow the same instructions as for Salamba Sarvangasana.

RELATED POSE. Halasana

ANANTASANA WITH A BOLSTER
SIDE-LYING LEG STRETCH

8.22
*Anantasana
with a Bolster*

PROPS
• 1 nonskid mat
• 1 bolster

OPTIONAL PROPS
• 1 blanket
• 1 strap

This variation of Anantasana with a Bolster (Figure 8.22) is recommended as a counterpose after practicing Salamba Sarvangasana (Figure 8.21) and Halasana (Figure 3.17) because it opens the hips, relaxes the shoulders, and lengthens the neck.

Place a bolster lengthwise on a nonskid mat. Then lie on your right side with the bolster supporting your right buttock and the right side of your back. (If you do not have a bolster, use a rolled blanket instead.) Extend your right arm overhead in line with your spine. Then bend your right elbow and rest the base of your skull in the palm of your right hand with your fingers supporting your neck. With an inhalation, bend your left knee and take hold of the big toe of your left foot with the second and third fingers of your left hand. With an exhalation, straighten your left leg and extend your left arm. (If your hamstrings are tight, use a strap around your left foot.)

In Anantasana with a Bolster, check that your inner groins are in line with your kidneys. Then firm your inner right calf, and lengthen your right kidney away from your right inner groin. At the same time, lengthen from your outer right armpit to your inner right elbow, and tuck your chin toward your left collarbone. With the palm of your right hand, lift the base of your skull away from the back of your neck to release and lengthen your cervical spine. Then lengthen from your outer left armpit to your inner left elbow, and draw the spine of C7 toward the spine of T1.

Maintain this position for 1 minute. Draw the spine of C7 toward the spine of T1, the spine of T1 toward the spine of T2, and the spine of T2 toward the spine of T3. Turn your chin toward your left collarbone, and lift the base of your skull away from the back of your neck to lengthen your cervical spine.

To come out of the pose, with an inhalation, bend your left knee and lower your left foot; with an exhalation, extend your left leg to meet your right leg. Then repeat to the other side.

PASCHIMOTTANASANA
SITTING FORWARD BEND

PROPS
- 1 nonskid mat
- 1 blanket or wedge

OPTIONAL PROPS
- 2 blocks
- 1 chair

8.23a
*Paschimottanasana,
Phase 1*

This variation of Paschimottanasana has an active and a restorative phase. In the active phase (Figure 8.23a), your head is raised to strengthen the muscles at the base

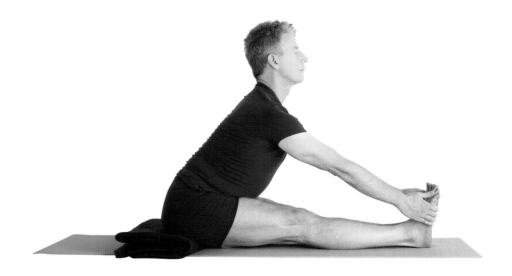

of your neck and lengthen your spine. In the restorative phase (Figure 8.23b), your head is lowered, your spine is relaxed, and you move deeper into the pose.

Place a folded blanket or wedge on your mat. Then sit at the edge of the blanket or wedge with your legs extended. Bend your elbows and place your fingertips on the floor behind your pelvis. Lift your kidneys away from your inner groins and broaden your midsternum. Then widen your collarbones, turn your sternal notch toward the base of your throat, and let your head drop back. With an inhalation, raise your arms overhead and draw the spine of C7 toward the spine of T1. With an exhalation, extend your torso over your thighs and take hold of your feet. (If you cannot reach your feet easily, use two blocks or the seat of a chair to support your hands.)

Phase 1. In Paschimottanasana, draw your inner groins away from your kidneys, and let your kidneys soften and sink deeper into your body. Widen your midthoracic vertebrae, so that you are not tempted to pull your lower spine forward. With an inhalation, lift your head from the base of your skull, and draw the spine of C7 toward the spine of TI, the spine of T1 toward the spine of T2, and the spine of T2 toward the spine of T3. Feel how the action of your upper thoracic spine helps to release tension from the front edge of your respiratory diaphragm.

Phase 2. With a deep exhalation, bend your elbows out to the side, and lower your chin toward your sternal notch. Maintain this position for 1 to 2 minutes. Relax your shoulders and widen the muscles at the base of your neck. Press the nodes of your upper back into your rib cage, and lengthen your upper arms toward your elbows. Turn the spine of C7 away from the spine of T1 to relax your upper thoracic spine. Then widen your sternal notch, and release the base of your skull away from your cervical spine.

To come out of the pose, raise your head from the base of your skull and straighten your arms. With an inhalation, draw the spine of C7 toward the spine of T1 as you raise your arms overhead and return to an upright position. With an exhalation, turn your palms out and lower your arms.

8.23b
Paschimottanasana, Phase 2

RELATED POSES. Janu Sirsasana, other sitting forward bends

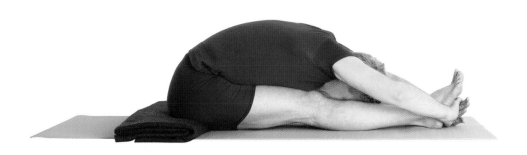

UJJAYI PRANAYAMA SITTING
BASIC YOGA BREATHING

PROPS	OPTIONAL PROPS
• 1 nonskid mat	• 1 or 2 blocks or blankets
• 1 blanket	• 1 wedge

This variation of Ujjayi Pranayama Sitting focuses on proper alignment of the upper thoracic and cervical spines to release the head and neck, relieve tension at the base of the throat, and deepen the chin lock.

Rest in Savasana (Figure 3.22) for 2 to 3 minutes before you begin your breathing practice. Then sit on your mat at the edge of a folded blanket in your most comfortable sitting position: Padmasana (Lotus Pose, Figure 3.21), Siddhasana (Perfect Pose, Figure 4.24), Sukhasana (Easy Pose, Figure 6.22), or Virasana (Hero Pose, Figure 5.24). If your knees are not in contact with the floor, use blocks or blankets to support them. (If you find it helpful, place the thin edge of a wedge under your sitting bones to give an additional lift to your pelvis and spine.)

8.24
Siddhasana

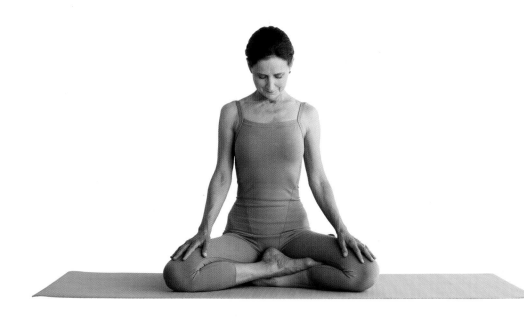

Bring your elbows to the sides of your waist, so that the backs of your arms are in line with your upper back, and rest the palms of your hands on your thighs. Lift the base of your skull toward the crown of your head as you drop your chin toward your upper sternum. Close your eyes gently and draw your eyes deep into their sockets.

Begin with a deep, soft exhalation. With each inhalation, lift your kidneys away from your inner groins, firm your inner elbows as you press the nodes of your upper back into your body, and draw the spine of T2 away from the spine of T1. At the same time, lift the spine of C7 away from the spine of T1 and widen your sternal notch. Keep your eyes soft. With each exhalation, keep the nodes of your upper back firm to stabilize your spine, and let your groins move away from your kidneys. Repeat this cycle for 3 to 5 minutes. Then let your breath return to normal, raise your head, change the cross of your legs, and repeat for another 3 to 5 minutes.

SAVASANA WITH SUPPORT UNDER C7
RELAXATION POSE VARIATION

PROPS
- 1 nonskid mat
- 1 facecloth

OPTIONAL PROP
- 1 blanket

In this variation of Savasana with Support Under C7 (Figure 8.25), a folded facecloth placed under the base of your neck helps to lift your C7 away from the floor and allows your shoulders to relax and descend.

Take a facecloth and fold it in quarters; then fold it again in thirds. Lie on your back on your mat or blanket. Place the folded facecloth lengthwise so that it supports your spine from C6–C7 at the base of your neck to T3–T4 between your shoulder blades.

8.25
Savasana with Support Under C7

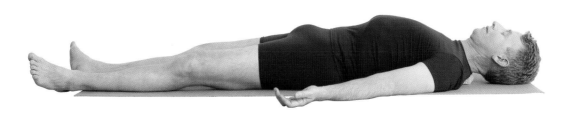

(If your chin tilts upward, place a folded blanket under your head to support the base of your skull.)

Now extend your arms and legs, and check the height and position of the support at the base of your neck. Adjust the height of the facecloth if it feels either too thick or too thin. Adjust the placement of the facecloth if it feels too high or too low on your upper thoracic spine. When you have found the best position for the facecloth, extend your arms and relax your shoulders. Move the base of your skull away from the back of your neck and gently close your eyes. Remain in this position for 5 to 10 minutes, observing the flow of the breath in your upper chest.

Practice Notes. If the support under the base of your neck is not helpful, here is a way to adjust your neck in Savasana without using the facecloth.

Lie on your back with your knees bent and your feet flat on the floor. Extend your arms by the sides of your body with your palms facing up. With an inhalation, lift your pelvis 1 or 2 inches off your mat, and press your upper thoracic spine into the floor. With an exhalation, move the base of your skull away from the back of your neck and, at the same time, turn the spine of C7 toward the spine of T1.

With another inhalation, widen your collarbones and relax your shoulders. With an exhalation, move the base of your skull away from the back of your neck, and turn the spine of T1 toward the spine of T2. Relax the sides of your neck, and allow your cervical spine to lengthen. Then lower your pelvis to the floor; extend your legs, one at a time; and remain in Savasana for 5 to 10 minutes.

► PRACTICE SEQUENCE

TADASANA

VIRABHADRASANA II

ARDHA CHANDRASANA

UTTANASANA

UTTHITA TRIKONASANA

PARIVRTTA TRIKONASANA

PADANGUSTHASANA

VIRABHADRASANA I

ADHO MUKHA SVANASANA

PINCHA MAYURASANA AT THE WALL

USTRASANA

VIPARITA DANDASANA WITH FEET ON A CHAIR

BHARADVAJASANA II

SALAMBA SIRSASANA

SETU BANDHASANA WITH BLOCKS UNDER THE SACRUM

SALAMBA SARVANGASANA

HALASANA

ANANTASANA WITH A BOLSTER

PASCHIMOTTANASANA

UJJAYI PRANAYAMA SITTING

SAVASANA WITH SUPPORT UNDER C7

GLOSSARY

Acromio-clavicular joint. The joint formed by the outer corner of the collarbone and the acromion process of the shoulder blade (Figure 6.1).

Anterior superior iliac spine. The boney angle formed by the front, or anterior, hipbone and the top, or crest, of the hipbone.

Asana. Yoga pose or poses.

C1–C7. The seven cervical vertebrae are labeled C1–C7, from upper to lower (Figure 8.4).

C7. The seventh cervical vertebra marks the critical junction between the cervical spine and the thoracic spine, and is characterized by a prominent spinous process (Figure 8.4).

Cervical spine. The seven vertebrae, or bones, of the neck (Figure 8.4).

Coccyx. The tailbone.

Eyes of the chest. The hollows of the upper chest, located between the upper ribs and the lower edge of the collarbones (Figure 4.3).

Floating ribs. The lower ribs, not directly attached to the sternal body.

Glenoid cavity. The outer corner, or lateral angle, of the shoulder blade that forms part of the shoulder joint (Figure 6.1).

Groins. The muscles and ligaments of the front hip crease, where the thighs join the pelvis.

Humerus. The upper arm bone.

Hyaline cartilage. A translucent kind of cartilage, present in joints and the respiratory tract, and forming much of the fetal skeleton.

Iliacus. This muscle originates from the interior wall of the hipbone (ilium), merges with the psoas, and inserts on the lesser trochanter of the thighbone (Figure 5.1).

Iliopsoas. The iliacus and psoas are sometimes referred to as the iliopsoas because they generally function together as a single unit (Figure 5.1).

Iyengar-style yoga. The practice of hatha yoga based on the teachings of B. K. S. Iyengar, author of *Light on Yoga*.

Kyphosis. An outward curvature of the thoracic spine, causing a pronounced rounding of the upper back.

L1–L5. The five vertebrae that form the lumbar spine are labeled L1–L5, from upper to lower (Figure 8.4).

Lesser trochanter. The boney protruberance on the upper inner thighbone where the iliopsoas inserts.

Lumbar-sacral joint. The joint formed by the fifth lumbar vertebra (L5) and the top edge of the sacrum.

Manubrium. The upper sternum (Figure 4.1).

Midsternum. The sternal body (Figure 4.1).

Nuchal ligament. The thick, elastic ligament supporting the nape, or back, of the neck.

Palate. The roof of the mouth.

Paraspinal muscles. The muscles that run lengthwise on either side of the spinal column.

Pelvic diaphragm. The floor of the pelvis that supports the abdominal organs and is involved in respiratory movement (Figure 3.1).

Psoas. The deep muscle of the abdomen that originates from the lumbar vertebrae, passes through the pelvis, and inserts on the lesser trochanter of the thighbone (Figure 5.1).

Quadriceps. The large muscle of the front thigh that straightens the knee and helps to flex the hip joints.

Respiratory diaphragm. The main diaphragm, or primary muscle of respiration, separates the abdominal cavity and the thoracic cavity (Figure 3.1).

Sacroiliac. The joint between the hipbone (ilium) and the sacrum.

Scapula, scapulae. Shoulder blade, shoulder blades (Figure 6.1).

Scoliosis. A lateral curvature of the spinal column.

Shoulder girdle. The shoulder girdle is formed by the shoulder blades, collarbones, and manubrium (Figure 5.4).

Spinous process. The bony projection at the back of each vertebral body, which can be felt under the surface of the skin (Figure 8.4).

Splenius. The deeper muscles of the neck, formed by the splenius capitis and splenius cervicus (Figure 8.2).

Sternal notch. The groove at the base of the throat between the inner corners of the collarbones (Figure 5.4).

Sterno-clavicular joint. The joint formed by the inner corner of the collarbone and the manubrium (Figure 5.4).

Sternum. The breastbone (Figure 5.4).

T1–T12. The twelve thoracic vertebrae are labeled T1–T12, from upper to lower (Figure 8.4).

Thoracic diaphragm. The layer of muscles and connective tissue that separates the thoracic cavity from the head and neck, also known as the thoracic inlet, is involved in respiratory movement (Figure 3.1).

Thoracic spine. The twelve vertebra of the upper back, each one connected to a pair of ribs (Figure 8.4).

Thoraco-lumbar joint. The junction of the thoracic spine and the lumbar spine.

Transverse process. The lateral projection on either side of each vertebral body.

Trapezius. The broad muscle of the upper back, shoulders, and neck (Figure 8.2).

Triceps. The muscles of the back upper arm that straighten the elbow and help to extend the arm. (Figure 7.4)

Xiphoid process. The protruberance, or tail, at the base of the sternal body (Figure 4.1).

RESOURCES

▶ YOGA WITH DONALD MOYER

Donald Moyer offers ongoing yoga classes and an Advanced Studies Program at The Yoga Room, Berkeley, California, as well as workshops throughout the United States. All are open to interested individuals, yoga teachers, and health care professionals. For more information, visit www.yogaroomberkeley.com or e-mail info@yogaroom berkeley.com.

▶ CHAIR, CLOTHING, AND PROPS PHOTOGRAPHED IN *YOGA: AWAKENING THE INNER BODY*

Chair: Meco Corporation, (800) 251-7558, www.meco.net

Clothing: Marie Wright Yoga Wear, (800) 217-0006, www.mariewright.com

Props: Hugger-Mugger Yoga Products, (800) 473-4888, www.huggermugger.com

ABOUT THE MODELS

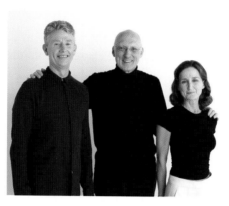

CANDACE CAREY SATLAK began her study of Iyengar-style yoga in 1984, and has been teaching since 1990. Joseph Satlak started his practice of Iyengar-style yoga in 1991, and has been teaching since 1995. They met while teaching at the B. K. S. Iyengar Yoga Center of Greater Boston, and are currently codirectors of the Belmont Yoga Studio in Belmont, Massachusetts. Candace and Joseph share an interest in macrobiotics and Vipassana meditation. They have been studying with Donald Moyer since 1992.

For information about classes at the Belmont Yoga Studio, visit www.belmontyoga.com. To e-mail Candace and Joseph, write to info@belmontyoga.com.

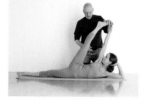

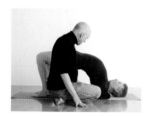

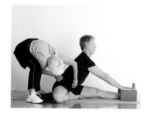

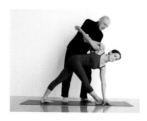

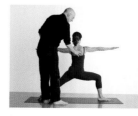

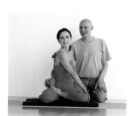

ABOUT THE AUTHOR

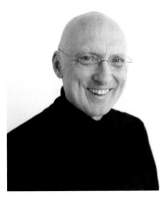

DONALD MOYER was born in Brooklyn, New York, in 1939. He was elected to Phi Beta Kappa at Cornell University in 1959, and received an Honours B.A. in English Language and Literature from Brasenose College, Oxford, in 1962. He worked as a computer programmer and systems analyst in London during the 1960s. In 1971, he took his first yoga class with Penny Nield-Smith at the Dance Center in Floral Street, just around the corner from the Royal Opera House in Covent Garden.

In 1974, Donald moved to Vancouver, British Columbia, where, with the help and support of Maureen Carruthers, he began teaching yoga. In January 1976, he studied for the first time with B. K. S. Iyengar as part of a group of ten or twelve students at the Ramamani Iyengar Memorial Yoga Institute in Pune, India. He returned to Pune frequently between 1976 and 1988.

At the end of 1976, Donald moved to San Francisco to continue his studies at the Institute for Yoga Teacher Education (now the Iyengar Yoga Institute of San Francisco). Before he graduated, he was invited to join the faculty. In 1978, he founded The Yoga Room in Berkeley, California, which he continues to direct.

Donald wrote the "Asana" column for *Yoga Journal* in 1987, 1989, and 1992. In 1988, he and Linda Cogozzo started Rodmell Press, for the purpose of publishing quality books on yoga, Buddhism, and aikido.

For information about classes at The Yoga Room, visit www.yogaroomberkeley.com. You can contact Donald at info@yogaroomberkeley.com.

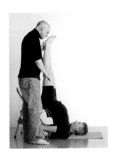
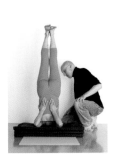
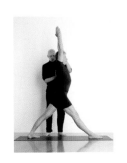
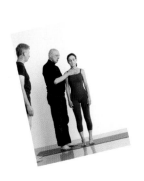
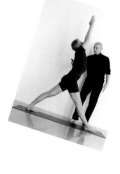

FROM THE PUBLISHER

RODMELL PRESS publishes books on yoga, Buddhism, and aikido. In the *Bhagavadgita* it is written, "Yoga is skill in action." It is our hope that our books will help individuals develop a more skillful practice—one that brings peace to their daily lives and to the earth.

We thank all whose support, encouragement, and practical advice sustain us in our efforts. In particular, we are grateful to Reb Anderson, B. K. S. Iyengar, Wendy Palmer, and Yvonne Rand for their inspiration.

To request a catalog or be on our e-announcements list, contact Rodmell Press:
(510) 841-3123 or (800) 841-3123
(510) 841-3191 (fax)
info@rodmellpress.com
www.rodmellpress.com

Rodmell Press is distributed to the trade by Publishers Group West:
(800) 788-3123
(510) 528-5511 (sales fax)
info@pgw.com

INDEX

Adho Mukha Svanasana
    collarbones, kidneys, and groins in, 122–123, 127–128
    diaphragms in, 65, 67–68
    elbow stabilization in, 189–190
    manubrium alignment and, 94
    shoulder blades in, 150, 154–155
    sternum alignment and, 98–99
    strengthening the neck, 216–217
    thoracic spines in, 206–207
Adho Mukha Svanasana with Forehead Support, 49, 51–52
Adho Mukha Svanasana with Hands on Blocks, 182–183
Adho Mukha Virasana with a Bolster, 87
Adho Mukha Virasana with Arms Extended, 67, 68, 127
Adho Mukha Vrksasana at the Wall, 76–77, 94, 164, 192–193
Anantasana with a Bolster, 225–226
anatomical body vs. physiological body, 3
Ardha Chandrasana, 72–73, 210–211
Ardha Sirsasana with Forearms on the Wall, 197
Ardha Uttanasana with Hands on the Wall, 181–182
armpits, 152
asthma, 26, 28, 49
awakening, forms of, 3–5

back pain or discomfort, 23, 24, 28, 49
backbends, 34, 59, 95, 164, 206–207
Bharadvajasana II, 166–167, 195–196, 221–222
blankets (props), 6
blocks (props), 7
bolster (prop), 6
breathing
    asthma or sinus problems, 26, 28, 49
    role of diaphragms in, 64, 65
    Ujjayi Pranayama Lying, 117, 144–145
    Ujjayi Pranayama Lying with Shoulder Blades Supported, 172–173
    Ujjayi Pranayama Resting, 87
    Ujjayi Pranayama Sitting, 88–89, 118, 146, 173–174, 201–202, 228–229
Bridge Pose. *See Setu Bandhasana variations*

C7 (seventh cervical vertebra). *See also strengthening the base of the neck*
    alignment crucial for, 16
    assessing neck curve and, 16–17
    finding, 16
    in Salamba Sarvangasana, 15
    Savasana with Support under C7, 229–230
    Setu Bandhasana with a Roll under C7, 24, 27–28
    sloping vs. square-set shoulders and, 15
    in Tadasana, 207
Camel Pose, 77–78, 105–106, 162–163, 218–219
carrying angle in the arms, 177
cervical vertebrae. *See* C7 (seventh cervical vertebra); neck; strengthening the base of the neck
chair (prop), 7
Child's Pose. *See Adho Mukha Virasana variations*
collarbones (clavicles). *See also collarbones, kidneys, and groins*
    asymmetrical poses and, 125
    lateral movement of, 125
    location of, 121
    manubrium attached to, 124
    in Marichyasana III, 125
    overview, 124–126
    rolling down, 125, 126
    rolling up, 125–126
    in Salamba Sirsasana, 42–43
    shoulder blades attached to, 149
    shoulders and misalignment of, 42–43, 125
    sternal notch, 123–124
    in Tadasana, 122, 125
    thoracic diaphragm attached to, 65
    vulnerability to injury, 124
collarbones, kidneys, and groins. *See also collarbones (clavicles); inner groins; kidneys*
    in Adho Mukha Svanasana, 122–123, 127–128
    in Halasana, 140–141
    in Janu Sirsasana, 143–144
    in Marichyasana III at the Wall, 141–142
    in Padangusthasana, 128, 129–130
    in Parivrtta Trikonasana, 132–133

    in Parivrtta Uttanasana, 136–137
    in Paschimottanasana, 128, 142–143
    in Pincha Mayurasana at the Wall, 133–134
    practice sequence, 147
    in Prasarita Padottanasana, 128
    in Salabhasana, 134–135
    in Salamba Sarvangasana, 139–140
    in Salamba Sirsasana, 137–138
    in Savasana, 147
    in Setu Bandhasana with Blocks and a Strap, 138–139
    in Tadasana, 126
    in Ujjayi Pranayama Sitting, 146
    in Urdhva Dhanurasana, 135–136
    in Uttanasana, 128, 131–132
    in Utthita Trikonasana, 128–129
    in Virabhadrasana I, 130–131

diaphragms. *See also specific diaphragms*
    in Adho Mukha Svanasana, 67–68
    in Adho Mukha Vrksasana at the Wall, 76–77
    in Ardha Chandrasana, 72–73
    balancing tone and quality of, 64
    benefits of adjusting, 65
    body divided vertically by, 63
    creating space vertically, 64
    defined, 63
    in Halasana, 83–84
    in Janu Sirsasana with Hands on Blocks, 85–86
    in Marichyasana III, 80–81
    in Padangusthasana, 70–71
    parallel alignment of, 63, 66
    in Parivrtta Ardha Chandrasana at the Wall, 73–75
    in Paschimottanasana with Hands on Blocks, 84–85
    practice sequence, 91
    in Salamba Sarvangasana, 82–83
    in Salamba Sirsasana, 81–82
    in Savasana, 89–90
    in Tadasana, 63, 64, 65, 66
    in Ujjayi Pranayama Resting, 87
    in Ujjayi Pranayama Sitting, 88–89
    in Urdhva Dhanurasana, 79–80
    in Ustrasana, 77–78
    in Uttanasana, 71–72
    in Utthita Parsvakonasana, 68–69
    in Virabhadrasana I, 75–76

visualizing, 63, 64, 65
widening, 63–64
discomfort. *See* neck discomfort; pain or discomfort
Downward-Facing Dog Pose. *See* Adho Mukha Svanasana *and variations*

Eagle Pose Variation, 114–115
Easy Pose, 88, 118, 146, 173, 201, 228
ego vs. self, 4–5
Elbow Balance. *See* Pincha Mayurasana at the Wall
elbow stabilization
 in Adho Mukha Svanasana, 189–190
 in Adho Mukha Svanasana with Hands on Blocks, 182–183
 in Adho Mukha Vrksasana at the Wall, 192–193
 in Ardha Sirsasana with Forearms on the Wall, 197
 in Ardha Uttanasana with Hands on the Wall, 181–182
 balancing inner and outer triceps for, 178–179
 in Bharadvajasana II, 195–196
 carrying angle and, 177
 locking elbows and, 177
 narrowing elbow joint for, 178
 in Padangusthasana, 187–188
 in Paschimottanasana with Hands on Blocks, 200
 practice sequence, 203
 in Salamba Sarvangasana, 199
 in Salamba Sirsasana, 198
 in Savasana with Arms Supported, 201
 in Tadasana, 178, 179–180
 in Ujjayi Pranayama Sitting, 201–202
 in Urdhva Dhanurasana with Hands on a Wedge, 194–195
 in Urdhva Hastasana I, 180–181
 in Urdhva Mukha Svanasana, 193–194
 in Uttanasana with Hands on a Block, 185–186
 in Utthita Parsvakonasana with a Block, 186–187
 in Vasisthasana, 190–192
 in Virabhadrasana I, 188–189
 in Virabhadrasana II, 183–184
energizing poses, 13, 28, 29
enlightenment, 4–5
Extended Side-Angle Pose. *See* Utthita Parsvakonasana *and variations*
Extended Triangle Pose, 128–129, 155–156, 212–213
eyes of the chest, 94–95

facecloth (prop), 7, 14
fatigue, poses for reducing, 28, 29, 31, 33, 49
folded blankets (props), 6
Foster, Susan Leigh, xi–xii
Freedom from the Known (Krishnamurti), 4–5

Garudasana for Arms Only, 114–115
Griffin, John Lyndon, 205
groins. *See* collarbones, kidneys, and groins; inner groins

Halasana, 83–84, 113, 140–141, 169–170
Halasana with a Strap, 17–18
Half Headstand, 197
Half-Moon Pose, 72–73, 210–211
hand towels (props), 7, 14
Handstand, 76–77, 94, 164, 192–193
headaches, 24, 26, 28, 49
Head-of-the-Knee Pose. *See* Janu Sirsasana *and variations*
Headstand. *See* Salamba Sirsasana *and variations*
Hero Pose, 88, 118, 146, 173, 201, 228
high blood pressure, 24, 28, 49, 52

iliacus muscles, 121–122
illness, recovery from
 Adho Mukha Svanasana with Forehead Support for, 49
 Salamba Sarvangasana for, 13
 Salamba Sarvangasana with Feet on the Wall for, 31, 33
 Salamba Sirsasana and, 49
 Sarvangasana with a Chair for, 29
 Viparita Karani for, 28
inner body
 awakening of, 4–5
 as deeper muscles, 3
 as physiological body, 3–4
 as reflective mind, 4
 as self, 4
inner groins. *See also* collarbones, kidneys, and groins
 asymmetrical poses and, 122
 exercise for familiarizing yourself with, 122
 kidneys and, 122–123
 location of, 121
 outer groins vs., 121
 overview, 121–122
 pelvis alignment and, 122
 in Utthita Parsvakonasana, 122
inverted poses, 34, 52–53, 164
Inverted Staff Pose, 219–220
Iyengar, B. K. S., xii, 1–3, 10, 93

Janu Sirsasana, 143–144
Janu Sirsasana with Hands on Blocks, 85–86, 115–116, 170–171

kidneys. *See also* collarbones, kidneys, and groins
 caution for moving, 124
 inner groins and, 122–123
 location of, 121, 122
 movement of, 122–124
 rib cage alignment with, 123
 in Salamba Sarvangasana, 21

Ujjayi Pranayama Lying for increasing awareness, 144–145
Krishnamurti, J., 4–5
kyphosis, 56

locking elbows, 177
Locust Pose, 134–135
Lotus Pose. *See* Padmasana *and variations*

manubrium (upper sternum). *See also* sternum
 anatomy of, 93
 checking alignment in mirror, 94
 collarbones attached to, 124
 eyes of the chest and, 94–95
 lifting the sternum and, 94
 posture and, 94
 rib cage shape and, 97
Marichyasana III, 80–81, 108–109, 125
Marichyasana III at the Wall, 141–142
mats, nonskid (prop)
 about, 6
 hair sticking to, 14
 neck roll using, 26
menstruation, poses to avoid during, 24, 49
midsternum (sternal body), 93, 94. *See also* sternum
migraines, 24, 26, 28, 49
mind, active vs. reflective, 4
Mountain Pose. *See* Tadasana *and variations*
Mountain Pose with Arms Overhead, 152, 180–181
Moyer, Donald, xi–xii, 1–3
muscles, surface vs. deeper, 3

neck. *See also* C7 (seventh cervical vertebra); strengthening the base of the neck
 assessing curve of, 16–17
 Savasana with a Neck Roll benefits for, 26
neck discomfort
 in Pincha Mayurasana at the Wall, 218
 in Salamba Sirsasana, 49–50, 58
 in Savasana with a Neck Roll, 26
 in Ustrasana, 219
 in Utthita Trikonasana, 128
neck injury
 manubrium alignment and, 94
 Salamba Sarvangasana alternatives and, 24
 Salamba Sirsasana alternatives and, 49, 52
 Sarvangasana with a Chair for recovery, 29
 Setu Bandhasana with a Roll under C7 and, 27
 Ustrasana and, 106
 Utthita Trikonasana and, 213

Nield-Smith, Penny, 1
nonskid mats. *See* mats, nonskid (prop)

operculum. *See* thoracic diaphragm

Padangusthasana
    collarbones, kidneys, and groins in,
        128, 129–130
    diaphragms in, 70–71
    elbow stabilization in, 187–188
    shoulder blades in, 158–159
    sternum alignment in, 100–101
    strengthening the neck, 214–215
Padmasana, 88, 118, 146, 173, 228
Padmasana with Hands on a Wedge, 201
pain or discomfort. *See also* neck dis-
        comfort
    approach to yoga and, xii
    back, 23, 24, 28, 49
    not persisting in, 9–10
    in Salamba Sirsasana, 58
Parivrtta Ardha Chandrasana at the Wall,
        73–75
Parivrtta Trikonasana, 103–104,
        132–133, 160–161, 213–214
Parivrtta Uttanasana, 136–137
Paschimottanasana, 128, 142–143,
        226–227
Paschimottanasana with Hands on
        Blocks, 84–85, 200
pelvic diaphragm. *See also* diaphragms
    aligning with other diaphragms, 63
    alignment of pelvis and, 64–65
    balancing with other diaphragms, 64
    body divided vertically by, 63
    coccyx and, 94
    overview, 64–65
    role in breathing, 64
    in Ujjayi Pranayama Resting, 87
    visualizing, 63, 64
    widening, overview, 63, 64
pelvis. *See also* pelvic diaphragm
    alignment, 64–65, 122
    sacrum, 94
    in Salamba Sarvangasana, 15, 22–23
    in Salamba Sirsasana, 47–48
Perfect Pose, 88, 118, 146, 173, 201, 228
physiological body vs. anatomical body,
        3
Pincha Mayurasana at the Wall
    collarbones, kidneys, and groins in,
        133–134
    shoulder blades in, 161–162
    sternum alignment in, 109–110
    strengthening the neck, 217–218
    Urdhva Hastasana II as preparation
        for, 164
Plough Pose. *See* Halasana *and variations*
Pose of Sage Marichi III. *See*
        Marichyasana III *and variations*
practice sequences. *See* sequencing poses
pranayama. *See* breathing

Prasarita Padottanasana, 49, 52–54, 128
props, 5–7, 9
psoas muscles, 121–122

Relaxation Pose. *See* Savasana *and varia-
        tions*
respiratory ailments
    asthma or sinus problems, 26, 28, 49
    Viparita Karani for, 28
respiratory diaphragm. *See also*
        diaphragms
    aligning with other diaphragms, 63
    balancing with other diaphragms, 64
    body divided vertically by, 63
    overview, 65
    role in breathing, 64, 65
    visualizing, 63, 65
    widening, overview, 63–64
    xiphoid process and, 94
retina, detached, 49
Revolved Half-Moon Pose, 73–75
Revolved Standing Forward Bend,
        136–137
Revolved Triangle Pose, 103–104,
        132–133, 160–161, 213–214
Right Angle Pose, 181–182
round bolster (prop), 6

sacrum, sternum compared to, 93–94
Salabhasana, 134–135
Salamba Sarvangasana, 12–35
    advice for beginners, 25
    assessing the neck curve, 16–17
    back discomfort in, 23
    balancing front and back body, 21
    balancing right and left sides, 19
    balancing the spine, 23–24
    balancing upper and lower body, 22
    blankets for, 13–15, 19–20, 33–34
    cautions and considerations, 24
    checking your alignment, 19–24
    collarbones, kidneys, and groins in,
        139–140
    coming into, 17–19
    defined, 13
    diaphragms in, 82–83
    elbow stabilization in, 199
    elbows, weight on, 14, 21, 22
    establishing foundation, 13–15
    hands on back, 18–19
    hands, pushing with, 22
    head, supporting, 14
    kidneys, adjusting, 21
    legs in, 21, 22–23
    lift under one elbow, 20
    manubrium alignment and, 94
    as mother of all poses, 37
    name explained, 13
    pelvis in, 15, 22–23
    practice notes, 33–34, 112
    pressure on C7, avoiding, 15
    rib cage, checking, 22

    Salamba Sirsasana and, 34, 59
    sequencing, 34–35, 59, 91, 119, 147,
        203, 231
    shoulder blades in, 150, 168
    shoulders in, 14–15, 20, 21, 22
    sternum alignment, 112
    strap on arms with, 17–18
    strengthening the neck, 224–225
    timing, 33
    variations and alternatives, 24, 25–33
Salamba Sarvangasana with Feet on the
        Wall, 25, 31–33
Salamba Sirsasana, 36–59
    advice for beginners, 41, 50
    arm length and, 37
    balancing front and back body, 43–46
    balancing right and left sides, 42
    balancing the spine, 48
    balancing upper and lower body,
        46–48
    cautions and considerations, 49–50, 58
    checking your alignment, 42–43
    collarbones, kidneys, and groins in,
        137–138
    collarbones level in, 42–43
    coming down from, 48–49
    coming into, 39–42
    diaphragms in, 81–82
    discomfort in, 58
    elbows in, 39, 42, 45–46, 198
    establishing foundation, 37–38
    as father of all poses, 37
    feet, thump coming down and, 49
    forearms in, 38, 40
    gaze, softening, 40–41
    hands in, 39, 40, 44–45
    head in, 38, 40, 41, 42, 43–45
    interlocking fingers, 39
    legs in, 41–42, 43, 46–49
    manubrium alignment and, 94
    pelvis alignment, 47–48
    physiological effects, 57–58
    practice notes, 57–58
    rib cage, checking, 46
    Salamba Sarvangasana and, 34, 59
    sequencing, 34, 58–59, 91, 119, 147,
        203, 231
    shoulder blades in, 46, 150, 167
    shoulders, adjusting, 42–43, 46
    sternum alignment in, 111
    strengthening the neck, 222–223
    timing, 57
    Urdhva Hastasana II as preparation
        for, 164
    variations and alternatives, 49, 51–57
    wrists in, 40, 45–46
Salamba Sirsasana at the Wall, 49, 50, 54,
        55
Salamba Sirsasana near the Wall, 50, 55
Salamba Sirsasana with Blocks at the
        Wall, 49, 56–57
samadhi, 4–5

Sarvangasana with a Chair, 24, 25, 29–31
Savasana, 89–90, 118–119, 147, 174–175
Savasana with a Neck Roll, 24, 25–26
Savasana with Arms Supported, 201
Savasana with Support under C7,
     229–230
scapulae. *See* shoulder blades
scoliosis
     Paschimottanasana and, 143
     Salamba Sarvangasana alternatives for,
          24
     Salamba Sirsasana and, 49
     Salamba Sirsasana with Blocks at the
          Wall and, 49, 56
     Sarvangasana with a Chair and, 29
self vs. ego, 4–5
sequencing poses
     for collarbones, kidneys, and groins,
          147
     for elbow stabilization, 203
     Salamba Sarvangasana, 34–35
     Salamba Sirsasana, 58–59
     for shoulder blades alignment, 175
     for sternum balancing, 119
     to strengthen the neck, 231
     for three diaphragms, 91
Setu Bandhasana with a Roll under C7,
     24, 27–28
Setu Bandhasana with Blocks and a
     Strap, 138–139
Setu Bandhasana with Blocks under the
     Sacrum, 223–224
seventh cervical vertebra. *See* C7 (sev-
     enth cervical vertebra)
shoulder blades. *See also* shoulders
     in Adho Mukha Svanasana, 150,
          154–155
     arms overhead and, 152–153
     in Bharadvajasana II, 166–167
     circular movement of, 152–153
     collarbones attached to, 149
     defined, 149
     dual function of, 149
     in Halasana, 169–170
     inferior, superior, and lateral angles,
          149
     in Janu Sirsasana with Hands on
          Blocks, 170–171
     medial, superior, and lateral borders,
          149
     in Padangusthasana, 158–159
     in Parivrtta Trikonasana, 160–161
     in Pincha Mayurasana at the Wall,
          161–162
     practice sequence, 175
     in Salamba Sarvangasana, 150, 168
     in Salamba Sirsasana, 46, 150, 167
     in Savasana, 174–175
     steps for adjusting, 149–152
     in Tadasana, 149, 150, 151–152, 153
     in Ujjayi Pranayama Lying with Shoul-
          der Blades Supported, 172–173

     in Ujjayi Pranayama Sitting, 173–174
     in Urdhva Dhanurasana, 165–166
     in Urdhva Hastasana I, 152
     in Urdhva Hastasana II, 163–164
     in Urdhva Mukha Svanasana, 150
     in Ustrasana, 162–163
     in Uttanasana, 156–157
     in Utthita Trikonasana, 155–156
     in Virabhadrasana I, 157–158
shoulders. *See also* shoulder blades
     collarbone misalignment and, 42–43,
          125
     injury, Salamba Sirsasana alternatives
          for, 52
     manubrium and, 94
     in Salamba Sarvangasana, 14–15, 20,
          21, 22
     in Salamba Sirsasana, 42–43, 46
     Sarvangasana with a Chair for relax-
          ing, 29
     sloping vs. square-set, 14–15
     widening, narrowing neck muscles
          and, 206
Shoulderstand. *See* Salamba Sarvan-
          gasana *and variations*
Siddhasana, 88, 118, 146, 173, 201, 228
Side Plank Pose, 190–192
Side-Lying Leg Stretch, 225–226
Simple Seated Twist II, 166–167,
          195–196, 221–222
sinus problems, 26, 28, 49
Sitting Forward Bend. *See* Paschimot-
          tanasana *and variations*
sitting forward bends, 34–35, 59, 95
sitting twists, 34–35, 59
slantboard or wedge (prop), 7
spine. *See also specific vertebrae*
     kyphosis, 56
     in Salamba Sarvangasana, 23–24
     in Salamba Sirsasana, 48
     scoliosis, 24, 29, 49, 56, 143
     spinous processes, 206–207
splenius muscles, 205–206, 207
standard folded blanket (prop), 6
Standing Forward Bend. *See* Uttanasana
     and variations
standing poses, 34, 58–59
sternal body (midsternum), 93, 94
sternum. *See also* manubrium (upper
     sternum); xiphoid process
     in Adho Mukha Svanasana, 98–99
     composite anatomy of, 93
     defined, 93
     in Garudasana for Arms Only,
          114–115
     in Halasana, 113
     in Janu Sirsasana with Hands on
          Blocks, 115–116
     as key to opening the chest, 93
     lifting, 93, 94
     in Marichyasana III, 108–109
     midsternum, 93, 94

     in Padangusthasana, 100–101
     in Parivrtta Trikonasana, 103–104
     in Pincha Mayurasana at the Wall,
          109–110
     practice sequence, 119
     sacrum compared to, 93–94
     in Salamba Sarvangasana, 112
     in Salamba Sirsasana, 111
     in Savasana, 118–119
     in Tadasana, 96
     in Tadasana with a Partner, 97
     in Ujjayi Pranayama Lying, 117
     in Ujjayi Pranayama Sitting, 118
     in Urdhva Dhanurasana, 107–108
     in Urdhva Mukha Svanasana, 104–105
     in Ustrasana, 105–106
     in Uttanasana, 102–103
     in Virabhadrasana I, 101–102
     in Virabhadrasana II, 99–100
strap (prop), 7
strengthening the base of the neck
     Adho Mukha Svanasana for, 216–217
     adjusting your cervical curve, 207
     Anantasana with a Bolster for,
          225–226
     Ardha Chandrasana for, 210–211
     Bharadvajasana II for, 221–222
     C7 as starting point for, 207
     cervical spine mirrored in thoracic
          spine, 207
     flat or concave upper back and, 207
     importance for neck protection, 206
     Padangusthasana for, 214–215
     Parivrtta Trikonasana for, 213–214
     Paschimottanasana for, 226–227
     Pincha Mayurasana at the Wall for,
          217–218
     practice sequence, 231
     rounded upper back and, 207
     Salamba Sarvangasana for, 224–225
     Salamba Sirsasana for, 222–223
     Savasana with Support under C7 for,
          229–230
     Setu Bandhasana with Blocks under
          the Sacrum for, 223–224
     Tadasana for, 208
     Ujjayi Pranayama Sitting for,
          228–229
     Ustrasana for, 218–219
     Uttanasana for, 211–212
     Utthita Trikonasana for, 212–213
     Viparita Dandasana with Feet on a
          Chair for, 219–220
     Virabhadrasana I for, 215–216
     Virabhadrasana II for, 209–210
     widening shoulders and narrowing the
          base of the neck, 206
stress, reducing, 28, 29
Sukhasana, 88, 118, 146, 173, 201, 228
Supine Mountain Pose with Arms
     Overhead, 163–164
Supported Shoulderstand, 24, 25, 28–29

Tadasana
    C7 in, 207
    collarbones, kidneys, and groins in, 122, 125, 126
    diaphragm alignments in, 63, 66
    elbow stabilization in, 178, 179–180
    finding C7 from, 16
    shoulder blades in, 149, 150, 151–152, 153
    sternum alignment in, 96
    strengthening the neck, 208
    thoracic spines in, 206–207
    visualizing diaphragms in, 63, 64, 65
Tadasana with a Partner, 97
tennis ball (prop), 7
tension, reducing, 28, 29
thoracic diaphragm. *See also* diaphragms
    in Adho Mukha Svanasana, 65
    aligning with other diaphragms, 63
    balancing with other diaphragms, 64
    body divided vertically by, 63
    overview, 65
    role in breathing, 64
    visualizing, 63, 65
    widening, 64
thoracic vertebrae. *See also* strengthening the base of the neck
    cervical vertebrae as mirror image of, 207
    distinguishing T1 from C7, 16
    injury, Setu Bandhasana with a Roll under C7 and, 27
    kyphosis, 56
    in Salamba Sirsasana, 48
    in Setu Bandhasana with a Roll under C7, 28
    spinous processes, 206–207
    splenius muscles and, 205
    thoracic diaphragm attached to, 65
    upper back flat or concave and, 207
timer (prop), 7
Toe-Holding Pose. *See* Padangusthasana
trapezius muscles, 15, 17, 205, 206
triceps, inner vs. outer, 178–179

Ujjayi Pranayama Lying, 117, 144–145
Ujjayi Pranayama Lying with Shoulder Blades Supported, 172–173, 175
Ujjayi Pranayama Resting, 87
Ujjayi Pranayama Sitting
    collarbones, kidneys, and groins in, 146
    diaphragms in, 88–89
    elbow stabilization in, 201–202
    shoulder blades in, 173–174
    sternum alignment and movement in, 118
    strengthening the neck, 228–229
Upward-Facing Bow Pose. *See* Urdhva Dhanurasana *and variations*
Upward-Facing Dog Pose, 104–105, 150, 193–194
Urdhva Dhanurasana
    collarbones, kidneys, and groins in, 135–136
    diaphragms in, 79–80
    shoulder blades in, 165–166
    sternum alignment in, 107–108
    Urdhva Hastasana II as preparation for, 164
Urdhva Dhanurasana with Hands on a Wedge, 194–195
Urdhva Hastasana I, 152, 180–181
Urdhva Hastasana II, 163–164
Urdhva Mukha Svanasana, 104–105, 150, 193–194
Ustrasana, 77–78, 105–106, 162–163, 218–219
Uttanasana
    collarbones, kidneys, and groins in, 123, 128, 131–132
    diaphragms in, 71–72
    Parivrtta Uttanasana with, 136, 137
    shoulder blades in, 156–157
    sternum alignment in, 102–103
    strengthening the neck, 211–212
Uttanasana with Hands on a Block, 185–186
Utthita Parsvakonasana, 68–69, 122
Utthita Parsvakonasana with a Block, 186–187

Utthita Trikonasana, 128–129, 155–156, 212–213

Vasisthasana, 190–192
Vasisthasana Facing a Wall, 191–192
Viparita Dandasana with Feet on a Chair, 164, 219–220
Viparita Karani, 24, 25, 28–29
Virabhadrasana I
    collarbones, kidneys, and groins in, 130–131
    diaphragms in, 65, 75–76
    elbow stabilization in, 188–189
    shoulder blades in, 157–158
    sternum alignment in, 101–102
    strengthening the neck, 215–216
Virabhadrasana II, 99–100, 183–184, 209–210
Virasana, 88, 118, 146, 173, 201, 228

Warrior Pose I. *See* Virabhadrasana I
Warrior Pose II, 99–100, 183–184, 209–210
wedge or slantboard (prop), 7
Wide-Leg Standing Forward Bend, 49, 52–54, 128

xiphoid process. *See also* sternum
    anatomy of, 93
    backbends and, 95
    defined, 65, 93
    forward bends and, 95
    respiratory diaphragm and, 65, 94
    sternum and spine coordinated by, 95
    tail of sacrum compared to, 94

Yoga: Awakening the Inner Body (Moyer)
    audience intended for, 5
    comparing poses in different chapters, xii
    overview, 8–9
    recommendations for using, 8, 9–10
    reinterpreting and carrying further, 10
yoga breathing. *See* breathing